SPANISH PROFICIENCY 2-IN-1 SERIES

SPANISH FOR ADULT BEGINNERS AND HEALTHCARE PROFESSIONALS: LEARN VOCABULARY AND MASTER PRONUNCIATION WITH EASE TO COMMUNICATE WITH ANYONE

SOL MANCILLA

CONTENTS

BOOK 1: LEARN SPANISH FOR ADULT BEGINNERS

BOOK 2: MEDICAL SPANISH FOR HEALTHCARE HEROES

BOOK 1: LEARN SPANISH FOR ADULT BEGINNERS

Learn Spanish for Adult Beginners

Speak Confidently & Impress Your Amigos
A No-Nonsense Guide to Quickly Learn
Vocabulary, Common Phrases, and Master
Pronunciation

Sol Mancilla

INTRODUCTION

Hola amigos! Have you ever been in a situation where you've found yourself completely lost in a conversation because of a language barrier? Maybe you thought you understood what was being said, only to realize later that you missed a key phrase or expression. This can be frustrating, embarrassing, and even comical at times. Trust me, I've been there!

Years ago, I was introducing some English friends to some Spanish friends, and we all attempted to have a conversation with the help of some translations. However, when one of my

Spanish friends used the expression "Donde Jesús perdió su merchero—Where Jesus lost his lighter—" (this phrase refers to a very remote and distant place), my English friends were completely lost. Their confused expressions made me realize that even the most basic phrases and expressions can be a challenge for someone learning a new language.

But fear not, my dear friends, for there is a solution! Learning a new language may seem intimidating, but it will also be one of the most rewarding experiences you can have. With the right tools and approach, you will gain a solid understanding of a new language and open doors to new cultures and experiences. That's why I'm excited to share with you my book, which will provide you with a fun and engaging way to learn Spanish. So, grab a cup of coffee, pull up a chair, and let's get started on this exciting journey together!

Maybe you need to learn Spanish for work and the pressure is blocking you from making any headway. Or perhaps you dream of traveling to Spanish-speaking countries but feel overwhelmed by all the vocabulary and grammar. It's okay, I understand your sorrow.

You're tired of old-school learning techniques like repeating a word over and over again. You want to learn different styles to improve your skills with a range of activities. You're probably thinking back to learning a language at school and how difficult it was. And now you're concerned about trying to understand different dialects and whether others will still understand you. You're constantly translating phrases, and the closest you've gotten to speaking Spanish is essentially a sitcom-styled "Spanglish."

But don't worry, I've got your back. This book is designed to help you overcome these common obstacles and learn Spanish with ease. You'll discover a whole new approach to learning that's engaging, practical, and most importantly, fun.

With my book, you'll gain a solid understanding of the foundations of Spanish, including a wide range of vocabulary, simple grammar rules, and sentence structure. Unlike other solutions, this book will challenge your brain in a fun way, leading to faster results and encouraging you to keep learning more. By the end of these pages, you'll feel certain about your understanding and have the confidence to start conversations with others, opening up a world of new opportunities.

So, whether you need Spanish for work or travel, this is the book for you. Say goodbye to frustration and hello to fluency!

As a language enthusiast, I know the struggle of trying to learn a new language. It can be daunting and frustrating, especially when you don't know where to start or how to continue. That's why I wrote this book: to be the catalyst that will trigger your desire to learn Spanish and provide you with the tools you need to succeed.

If you're reading this, chances are you're already aware of the benefits of learning Spanish. It's the second-largest language spoken by natives and the fourth most spoken language in the world. Being able to speak Spanish allows you to communicate with millions of people, both in your own community and around the world. You could unlock a whole new world of opportunities—from traveling to Spanish-speaking countries and experiencing their culture firsthand, to building new relationships and connections with people from different backgrounds.

But let's face it, learning a language is not easy. It takes dedication, patience, and a lot of hard work. That's where this book comes in. I want to make learning Spanish fun and enjoyable, rather than a chore. With a focus on practical conversation and real-world situations, you'll learn this wonderfully rich language and be able to use it in your everyday life.

No matter if you're a complete beginner or have some previous experience with Spanish, throughout these pages, I will provide you with a solid foundation of vocabulary, grammar, and sentence structure. And with a little bit of effort and practice, you'll soon be able to hold conversations with confidence and ease.

With my experience-proven methods and strategies, you'll be speaking Spanish in no time. No more tedious grammar drills or boring vocabulary lists. Instead, I offer a fun and engaging way to learn Spanish that will challenge your brain and make learning a breeze.

I've accumulated years of experience and knowledge to provide you with a solid understanding of the foundations of Spanish. And the best part? These methods are designed to help you learn faster! You won't be bogged down by lengthy explanations or confusing verb conjugations. Instead, I'll teach you the most essential aspects of the language that you need to know to start speaking with confidence.

This is not just about learning Spanish, it's about immersing yourself in the rich culture behind the language. You'll gain a deep appreciation for Spanish culture and be able to connect with Spanish-speaking communities in a meaningful way.

Now, let me paint a vivid picture of the end result you will achieve by reading this book: Imagine confidently walking into a room full of Spanish-speaking individuals and not only being able to understand everything they're saying but also being able to hold a conversation with them. Think about the new connections and opportunities that would open up for you! From ordering food at a restaurant to making new friends on your next trip to a Spanish-speaking country, the possibilities are endless.

And who better to guide you on this journey than a native Spanish speaker, like myself? I have spent 20 years living in South America and have immersed myself in the regional differences in the language. I have a passion for teaching and helping others gain the benefits of speaking two languages.

Think back to the days before the internet, before apps and language software, before easy access to foreign films and music. Learning a new language was a slow and frustrating process, and many people gave up before achieving any real proficiency.

But times have changed, and the new era of language learning is here. In this book, I'm going to reveal the secrets of how to learn

Spanish quickly and easily, without the frustration and confusion of traditional methods.

It wasn't always this easy. When I was first learning English, I struggled to make sense of the complex grammar and pronunciation rules. I felt like I was making no progress, and I was beginning to think that I would never be able to speak the language fluently.

But then, I discovered some new techniques and resources that changed everything. I learned how to focus on the most important vocabulary and grammar structures, how to immerse myself in the language and culture, and how to practice speaking with native speakers.

Now, I'm excited to share these techniques with you. With this book, you'll be able to achieve the promised result of speaking Spanish fluently and confidently. You'll learn how to pronounce every word, how to use practical vocabulary and phrases for everyday communication, and how to appreciate the prosperous and astonishing culture of Spanish-speaking countries.

So, don't give up on your dream of learning Spanish. The new era of language learning is here, and it's easier and more accessible than ever before. Let's get started—and soon enough you'll be ready to impress your amigos with your newfound Spanish skills!

¡Vamos a empezar!

THE SPANISH ALPHABET AND PRONUNCIATION

Are you ready to dive into the exciting world of Spanish? Before we start stringing words together to form sentences, we need to master the basics. One of the most fundamental aspects of learning Spanish is understanding the alphabet and how to pronounce each letter correctly.

The great news is that, unlike English, Spanish has a very consistent and logical system of pronunciation. Each letter is pronounced exactly as it is written, with no unexpected surprises or tricky letters to trip you up. So, let's get started on our journey to mastering the Spanish alphabet!

THE 27 LETTERS OF THE SPANISH ALPHABET

Firstly, it's important to know that the Spanish alphabet has the same 26 letters as the English alphabet, plus one additional letter, the ñ. This letter, which is pronounced "eh-nyeh," is used to represent a unique sound in the Spanish language.

To begin our journey, let's take a look at each letter of the Spanish alphabet and how to pronounce it correctly:

- **A** (ah): as in "hola (oh-lah)": hello
- **B** (beh): as in "baño (bah-nyoh)": bathroom
- **C** (ceh): as in "casa (kah-sah)": house
- **CH** (cheh): as in "mucho (moo-cho)": a lot/much
- **D** (deh): as in "deporte (deh-por-teh)": sport
- **E** (eh): as in "leche (leh-cheh)": milk
- **F** (eh-feh): as in "familia (fah-mee-lee-ah)": family
- **G** (heh): as in "gato (gah-toh)": cat
- **H** (a-cheh): as in "huevo (weh-boh)": egg
- **I** (ee): as in "isla (ee-slah)": island
- **J** (ho-tah): as in "jamón (hah-mohn)": ham
- **K** (kah): as in "karaoke (kah-rah-oh-keh)": karaoke
- **L** (eh-leh): as in "luna (loo-nah)": moon
- **LL** (eh-yeh): as in "llave (yah-beh)": key
- **M** (eh-meh): as in "manzana (mahn-sah-nah)": apple
- **N** (eh-neh): as in "nube (noo-beh)": cloud
- **Ñ** (eh-nyeh): as in "mañana (mah-nyah-nah)": morning
- **O** (oh): as in "hola (oh-lah)": hello
- **P** (peh): as in "perro (peh-roh)": dog
- **Q** (kuh): as in "queso (keh-soh)": cheese
- **R** (eh-reh): as in "ratón (rah-tohn)": mouse
- **RR** (eh-rreh): as in "arroz (ah-rrohz)": rice
- **S** (eh-seh): as in "sol (sohl)": sun
- **T** (teh): as in "tren (trehn)": train

- **U** (oo): as in "uno (oo-noh)": one
- **V** (oo-veh): as in "vaca (bah-kah)": cow
- **W** (doh-bleh veh): as in "wifi (wai-fai)": Wi-Fi
- **X** (eh-kees): as in "excusa (ehks-koo-sah)": excuse
- **Y** (yeh): as in "yogur (yoh-goor)": yogurt
- **Z** (zeh-tah): as in "zapato (sah-pah-toh)": shoe

You may have noticed that there are more than 27 letters in this list. That's because, in Spanish, there are 3 compound letters: "ch," "ll," and "rr." The first is known to English speakers in words like "chips" or "chain." We'll discuss "ll" and "rr" later on.

It's essential to take the time to learn and practice the correct pronunciation of each letter to build a strong foundation in Spanish. This will not only help you to pronounce words correctly but also make it easier to understand native Spanish speakers.

It is likely that simply by reading the name of these letters you are not using the correct pronunciation. Don't worry, it's normal. As an English speaker, your brain associates the letters you see with certain sounds. To learn Spanish—or any other language— you will have to build new associations between letters and sounds. I recommend that you check out this Busuu video, available on YouTube, which is super didactic and will help you understand the correct pronunciation of each letter in the Spanish alphabet: Spanish Alphabet: A Simple Guide for English Speakers

As a beginner, you may find Spanish pronunciation a bit challenging, but don't worry, I will make it easy for you to understand.

SYLLABLES AND SPANISH PRONUNCIATION RULES

One of the essential elements of Spanish pronunciation is syllables. In Spanish, most syllables end with a vowel: "ma-má" (mom), "pa-pe-les"(papers), and "a-mi-go" (friend).

Another important rule is that when there is a consonant between two vowels, it forms a syllable with the second vowel. For example, "ca-sa" (house), "pe-rro" (dog), "fa-mi-lia" (family).

It's also essential to understand the difference between strong and weak vowels. Strong vowels include "a," "e," and "o," while weak vowels include "i" and "u." When there is a combination of strong and weak vowels, the weak vowel will often blend in with the strong vowel. For example, "ai-re" (air), "hue-vo" (egg), and "mue-ble" (furniture).

Some consonants aren't separated, meaning they need to be pronounced together as one sound. These consonants include "ch," "ll," "rr," "gu," and "qu." For example, "cho-co-la-te," "lla-ma-da" (call), "a-rroz" (rice), "gue-rra" (war), and "que-so" (cheese).

When two consonants appear together, the first consonant is usually grouped with the preceding vowel, and the second consonant is grouped with the following vowel. For example, "planta" (plant) is divided into "plan-ta" and "apto" is "ap-to" (suitable).

For words with three or more consonants in a row, the rules become so complicated and tedious that most native Spanish speakers don't even know about them. But don't worry, over time you will develop the intuition necessary to separate into syllables, even without remembering the rules by heart. Don't worry about the meaning of the following list of words for now; some are quite advanced! Just focus on trying to learn how the words are separated by syllables.

Here, I leave you a list of words separated into syllables so that you become familiar with them:

- abstracto: abs-trac-to (abstract)
- abstraer: abs-tra-er (to abstract)
- substraer: subs-tra-er (to subtract)
- transplantar: trans-plan-tar (to transplant)
- demonstrar: de-mons-trar (to demonstrate)
- monstruo: mons-truo (monster)
- inscrutable: ins-cru-ta-ble (inscrutable)
- contracciones: con-trac-cio-nes (contractions)
- adscrito: ads-cri-to (assigned)
- circunscribir: cir-cuns-cri-bir (to circumscribe)

Lastly, it's important to understand that prefixes are syllables on their own. For example, "pre-his-tó-ri-co" (prehistoric), "pos-par-to" (postpartum), and "re-to-mar" (resume).

Let's explore the fascinating world of pronunciation in the Spanish language, where a set of rules govern the way words are spoken and sounds are produced. Understanding these rules is key to mastering the art of speaking Spanish fluently and accurately.

In Spanish, the letter "c" is pronounced differently depending on the vowel that follows it. When "c" is followed by an "a," "o," or "u," it is pronounced like the English "k" sound, as in the word "casa." However, when it is followed by an "e" or "i," it is pronounced like the English "s" sound, as in the word "celeste."

Let me show you some examples:

- cielo (cee-eh-loh): sky
- cámara (kah-mah-rah): camera
- césped (sehs-pehd): grass
- culpa (khul-pah): guilt
- correo (ko-rreh-oh): mail

Similarly, the letter "g" in Spanish has two different sounds. When "g" is followed by an "a," "o," or "u," it is pronounced like the English "g" sound, as in the word "gangster" or "gum." However, when "g" is followed by an "e" or "i," it is pronounced like the Spanish "j", with a stronger guttural sound, like imitating an angry kitty; or like a stronger English "h" in "hammer." Here you have some examples:

- goma (goh-mah): eraser
- gafas (gah-fahs): glasses
- gemelo (heh-meh-loh): twin
- gusto (guhs-toh): taste

When it comes to words that contain "gu," we must be careful since there are two special cases. If the "gu" is followed by an "e" or "i," the "u" won't be pronounced, but the "g" sound will still be soft. This rule also applies to many words in English like "guess" or "guillotine." Let me bring you some examples in Spanish:

- guitarra (ghee-tah-rrah): guitar
- guerra (gheh-rrah): war

It is important to mention that in Spanish, the "r" has a soft sound when it is between two vowels as well as at the end of words. For example: "pera" or "motor." In contrast, "r" has a rolling sound when it appears at the beginning of a word. For example: "rosa," "rompecabezas," or "roto." It is also pronounced rolling the "r" when it appears after the consonants "l", "n", and "s." For example: "alrededor" and "enredado."

Understanding these basic Spanish pronunciation rules will give you a strong base to build upon. Don't worry if it takes some time to master them. With practice and patience, you'll be on your way to speaking Spanish like a pro really soon!

UNDERSTANDING THE ACCENT

One of the most important aspects of speaking Spanish correctly is knowing how to use accents or tildes. These little lines over vowels are not just for decoration—they actually play a crucial role in conveying meaning. For example, the word "papá" (with an accent over the second a) means "dad," while "papa" (without the accent) means "potato." As you can see, accents can change the meaning of a word entirely, so it's important to know how to use them correctly.

To help you with this, here are **four rules for using Spanish tildes**:

- Tildes are used to indicate where the stress falls in a word. In general, if a word ends in a vowel, n, or s, the stress will fall on the next-to-last syllable. If it ends in any other letter, the stress will fall on the last syllable.
- Words that do not follow the above rule will have a tilde over the stressed vowel. For example, the word "árbol" (tree) has a tilde over the first syllable because that's where the stress falls.
- Tildes are used to distinguish between words that are spelled the same but have different meanings. For example, "si" means "if," while "sí" (with a tilde) means "yes."
- Finally, tildes are used in certain interrogative and exclamatory words to indicate emphasis. For example, "¡qué rico!" means "How delicious!"

By following these rules, you will be able to use accents correctly and avoid any confusion when speaking Spanish. So, practice these rules until you feel comfortable using them.

COMMON MISTAKES WITH SPANISH PRONUNCIATION

Let's now address some common mistakes that native English speakers make when pronouncing Spanish words. My experience taught me there are five common pronunciation errors, including mispronouncing the letter "r," pronouncing the letter "h" like the English "h," mispronouncing the letter "j," and confusing the pronunciation of "y" and "ll." These mistakes can often lead to confusion or even hilarity, as in the movie *Spanglish*, when Tea Leoni struggled with rolling the letter "r" while trying to say the name Flor.

- The rolling "r" sound is perhaps the most challenging for English speakers to master, but don't worry, with practice and patience, you'll get there! One tip is to place your tongue at the roof of your mouth and vibrate it as you exhale. It may feel awkward at first, but keep practicing, and you'll soon be rolling your "r"s like a native Spanish speaker.
- Unlike English, the letter "h" in Spanish is silent. That is, it has no sound. When a word contains "h," you just don't pronounce it. For example, "huevo" (egg), is pronounced "weh-boh."
- In Spanish, the letter "j" is pronounced differently than in English. It has a strong sound, similar to the "kh" sound in some Arabic or Hebrew words. This sound is created by forcefully pushing air through the back of the throat while holding the tongue freely without touching the roof of the mouth or teeth like you're about to spit. It's

important to note that the "j" sound in Spanish is not the same as the "h" sound, which is silent in Spanish. For instance, the word "jugo" (juice) is pronounced "hoo-goh."

- When learning Spanish, it's important to consider the pronunciation of "ll" and "y" as they can differ depending on the dialect. However, as a beginner, it may be best to focus on developing a neutral Spanish accent to ensure that you can communicate effectively with Spanish speakers from any country. In neutral Spanish, "ll" and "y" are pronounced the same way: as a soft "y" sound, similar to the "y" in the English word "yes." For example, the word "pollo," which means chicken, is pronounced "poh-yoh," and "playa" (beach) is pronounced "plah-yah."

5 TIPS TO SOUND MORE NATURAL

Pronunciation is one of the most challenging aspects of learning a new language. But with these **five tips**, you'll be well on your way to sounding more natural in no time:

1. **Focus on one Spanish accent/dialect:** Spanish is spoken in many countries and each country has its own unique accent and dialect. It's important to choose one accent/dialect that you like the most or that you'll be most likely to use in your daily life. For example, if you plan on visiting Mexico, then you should focus on Mexican Spanish. Same with Spain, Chile, and Argentina, since these three are among the most distinctive. This will help you become more comfortable with the sounds and intonations of that particular accent/dialect.

2. **Watch out for Bs and Vs:** In Spanish, the sounds for "B" and "V" are very similar, which can be confusing for non-native speakers. The key to mastering this is to practice, practice, practice! Listen closely to native speakers and try to mimic the way they pronounce these letters. The sound of the letter B is soft: "bueno" (good); instead, the letter V sounds louder, with a stricter sound, and with a tighter mouth: "valor" (value).

3. **Make an effort to pronounce accents:** Spanish is a language that uses accents to indicate where the emphasis falls in a word. It's important to pay attention to these accents and make an effort to pronounce them correctly. This will make your speech sound more natural and help you avoid misunderstandings.

4. **Practice with tongue twisters:** Tongue twisters are a fun and effective way to practice your pronunciation. They're challenging to say, but with practice, you'll start to master them. Here's an example: "Tres tristes tigres comen trigo en un trigal." The sound made up of a T and an R (tr) is particularly difficult for those who are not familiar with Spanish, so don't get frustrated if you don't make it at the beginning. Give it a shot, and keep trying!

5. **Link words together:** In Spanish, words often sound like they were linked together. It makes it difficult for non-native speakers to understand natives. However, by practicing this technique, you can make your speech sound more natural. For example, instead of saying "yo tengo hambre" (I am hungry), you can link the words together and say "yoten-goham-bre."

With so many resources available online, it can be tempting to rely on online translators to learn new words and phrases. However, while these tools provide an example of how to pronounce words, they don't offer a practical solution for retaining new vocabulary.

That's where a good old-fashioned notebook comes in handy. Writing down each new word and its corresponding phonetic pronunciation in your own phonetic alphabet is a great way to ensure that the new vocabulary stays in your brain. For example, the Spanish word "lluvia" (rain) can sound like "youvia" to an English speaker. Writing it down in your notebook as "lluvia, rain /youvia/" will not only help you remember the word, but it will also aid in your pronunciation. Even better, you can also attach an image of rain so that your brain builds neural bridges and makes the correct associations between images, objects, words, and pronunciation.

Of course, it takes more effort than simply relying on an online translator, but the reward is worth it. By writing down each new word in your notebook, you're actively engaging your brain and committing the new vocabulary to memory. Plus, you'll have a handy reference guide to look back on when you need to recall a word or phrase.

With your trusty notebook in hand, it's time to dive into core vocabulary that will serve as the building blocks for communication. Whether you're learning Spanish for travel, work, or personal enrichment, it's important to start with the basics. From common greetings and expressions to essential verbs and adjectives, the more words you learn, the more confident you'll become in your ability to communicate in Spanish.

If you don't know how to spell it, ask a native speaker to help you with the proper spelling and pronunciation of the word or phrase. This way, you will gradually train your ear to recognize the words and the local speaking style. We Spanish speakers love it when others try to learn our language and we are happy to help them. So, don't be afraid to ask. I promise you that no one will make fun of you!

So, take the time to invest in your language-learning journey. By putting in the effort to write down new vocabulary in your notebook and regularly reviewing it, you'll be on your way to speaking Spanish with ease in no time.

To start incorporating the habit of learning Spanish into your daily life, you can implement some of these simple, fun, and effective didactic tasks. Time to do homework!

- **Make your home a Spanish classroom!** Label everything in your home with its Spanish name. This will help you learn new vocabulary every day without even realizing it. You can start with the kitchen: label the dishes, the cutlery, the utensils, the furniture, etc. The following week you can do the same with the objects in the bedroom, bathroom, and garden, among others.
- **Sing your way to Spanish fluency!** Sing along to Spanish songs and pay attention to the lyrics. This will help you improve your pronunciation and vocabulary. You can opt for slow songs to be able to identify the

pronunciations of the words while you hear and read them.

- **Netflix and learn:** Watch Spanish TV shows or movies with English subtitles. Pay attention to how the words sound and try to repeat them out loud.

PRACTICE AND VOCABULARY

1. **Separate the following words into syllables:**
2. Equívoco/a (ambiguous)
3. Análogo/a (analogous)
4. Disuadir (dissuade)
5. Estipulación (stipulation)
6. Evocar (evoke)
7. Frenético/a (frantic)
8. Indolencia (indolence)
9. Influir (influence)
10. Introspección (introspection)
11. Lúdico/a (ludic)
12. Mitigar (mitigate)
13. Paradoja (paradox)
14. Perspicaz (perspicacious)
15. Plausible (plausible)
16. Prejuicio (prejudice)
17. Procrastinar (procrastinate)
18. Propagación (propagation)
19. Recalcitrante (recalcitrant)
20. Resiliente (resilient)
21. Sarcástico/a (sarcastic)

22. Serendipia (serendipity)
23. Sobresaliente (outstanding)
24. Soslayar (bypass)
25. Trascendente (transcendent)
26. Volátil (volatile)

Answers:

1. e-quí-vo-co/a
2. a-ná-lo-go/a
3. di-sua-dir
4. es-ti-pu-la-ción
5. e-vo-car
6. fre-né-ti-co/a
7. in-do-len-cia
8. in-flu-ir
9. in-tros-pec-ción
10. lú-di-co/a
11. mi-ti-gar
12. pa-ra-do-ja
13. pers-pi-caz
14. plau-si-ble
15. pre-jui-cio
16. pro-cras-ti-nar
17. pro-pa-ga-ción
18. re-cal-ci-tran-te
19. re-si-lien-te
20. sar-cás-ti-co/a
21. se-ren-di-pia
22. so-bre-sa-lien-te

23. sos-la-yar
24. tras-cen-den-te
25. vo-lá-til

In Spanish, there are different rules for accentuating a word. The accent or tilde fulfills the function of indicating which is the syllable that is pronounced with more emphasis in a word. Since these rules are a bit complicated and beyond the comprehension of an amateur learner, we are going to skip learning them and instead, I will leave you a list of words with accents in Spanish so that you know them and develop an intuition about them:

- Árbol (tree): ahr-bohl
- Ídolo (idol): ee-doh-loh
- Época (epoch): eh-poh-kah
- Música (music): moo-see-kah
- Fácil (easy): fah-seel
- Útil (useful): oo-teel
- Así (like this, so): ah-see
- Camión (truck): kah-myohn
- Público (public): poo-blee-koh
- Página (page): pah-hee-nah
- Américas (Americas): ah-meh-rih-kahz
- Matemáticas (mathematics): mah-teh-mah-tee-kahs
- Sábado (Saturday): sah-bah-doh
- Único (unique): oo-nee-koh
- Pirámide (pyramid): pee-rah-mee-deh
- Grúa (crane): groo-ah
- Clímax (climax): klee-mahx
- Ejército (army): eh-hehr-see-toh

- Fantástico (fantastic): fahn-tahs-tee-koh
- Esquí (ski): ehs-kee
- Cálido (warm): kah-lee-doh
- Óptimo (optimal): ohp-tee-moh
- Víctima (victim): beek-tee-mah
- Mágico (magical): mah-hee-koh
- Cárcel (jail): kahr-sehl
- Médico (medical): meh-dee-koh
- Ácido (acid): ah-see-doh
- Apólogo (apologue): ah-poh-loh-goh
- Sónico (sonic): soh-nee-koh
- Antártida (Antarctica): ahn-tahr-tee-dah

ESSENTIAL SPANISH VOCABULARY

¿Hablas español? Spanish, in particular, is a language with a rich and complex history. From its roots in Latin to the influence of Arabic during the Middle Ages, Spanish has evolved into the magnificent language we know and love today.

The Spanish language is a fascinating and rich language that has an interesting history. The origins of this stunning language can be traced back to the Iberian Peninsula, where the Celtic and Iberian languages were spoken. The Roman Empire conquered the peninsula in the 3rd century BC, and Latin became the language of the land. Over time, Latin evolved into what we now know as Spanish.

Spanish has been greatly influenced by other cultures and languages. In the 8th century AD, the Moors, a Muslim people from North Africa, invaded the peninsula and brought with them the Arabic language. Arabic words can still be found in the Spanish language today. The word "ojala" serves as an example. It has evolved from the Arabic phrase "law šá lláh," which translates to "If god would want it" or "God willing." Today, the word has lost its religious connotation and is primarily used to express "I hope." People of different religions, including Catholics, Christians, Muslims, and atheists, use the word without realizing its origins (WhyNotSpanish, 2018).

As Spain expanded its territories through conquest and colonization in the 15th and 16th centuries, the Spanish language spread throughout the Americas, Africa, and Asia. This led to the emergence of various dialects, each with its own unique characteristics and nuances.

Today, Spanish is the second most spoken language in the world, with over 500 million speakers worldwide. It is the official language of Spain and many Latin American countries, as well as one of the official languages of the United Nations.

The expansion of Spanish has not only contributed to its linguistic influence but has also shaped the culture and identity of the regions where it is spoken. It has been an integral part of the development of literature, art, music, and cinema, and has helped to connect people across borders and cultures (Newsdle, n.d.).

But enough about history, let's get down to business: essential Spanish vocabulary. In this chapter, we will cover a wide range of vocabulary. But we won't just give you a list of words and their translations. We'll also provide you with contextualized examples.

One of the best ways to reinforce new vocabulary is through repetition and practice. That's why I've included exercises and activities to help you master the words you've learned. You'll also have the opportunity to practice your new vocabulary in the context of real-life situations, like ordering food in a restaurant or asking for directions on the street.

By the end of this chapter, you'll have a solid foundation of essential Spanish vocabulary and the confidence to use it in everyday situations. So, grab a pen and paper, and let's get started! ¡Vamos!

Are you ready to dive into the colorful world of Spanish vocabulary? Next, we're going to explore the vibrant and exciting world of colors and shapes. From the deep blue of the ocean to the bright red of a ripe tomato, we'll cover it all!

COLORS, SHAPES, AND SIZES

Here's a quick list of some essential colors in Spanish, their translations to English and their proper Spanish pronunciation:

- rojo (red): rroh-hoh
- azul (blue): ah-sool
- amarillo (yellow): ah-mah-ree-yoh
- naranja (orange): nah-rahng-hah
- verde (green): berh-deh
- morado (purple): moh-rah-doh
- rosado (pink): rrohh-sah-doh
- marrón (brown): mah-rrohn
- negro (black): neh-groh

- blanco (white): blahn-kho
- gris (gray): grees

Now, let's move on to the world of shapes and geometrical figures. I'll also provide you with plenty of opportunities to practice using these words so that they become second nature to you.

- cuadrado (square): kwah-drah-doh
- triángulo (triangle): tree-ahn-goo-loh
- rectángulo (rectangle): rehk-tahn-goo-loh
- círculo (circle): seehr-koo-loh
- elipse (ellipse): eh-leep-seh
- rombo (rhombus): rohm-boh
- trapecio (trapezoid): trah-peh-syoh
- pentágono (pentagon): pehn-tah-goh-noh
- hexágono (hexagon): ehks-ah-goh-noh
- estrella (star): ehs-treh-yah

Now, let's learn about sizes:

- pequeño (little): peh-keh-nyoh
- mediano (medium): meh-dee-ah-noh
- grande (big): grahn-deh

THE HUMAN BODY

Now, let's get started with some basic vocabulary related to the human body. After all, knowing how to describe body parts is not only useful for everyday conversations, but it can also be helpful in emergencies. So, let's start with some translations:

- cabeza (head): kah-beh-sah
- ojos (eyes): oh-hohs
- nariz (nose): nah-reez
- oreja (ear): oh-reh-hah
- boca (mouth): boh-kah
- lengua (tongue): lehn-gwah
- dientes (teeth): dee-ehn-tehs
- labios (lips): lah-bee-ohs
- garganta (throat): gahr-gahn-tah
- cuello (neck): kweh-yoh
- hombro (shoulder): ohm-broh
- espalda (back): ehs-pahl-dah
- pecho (chest): peh-choh
- brazo (arm): brah-soh
- codo (elbow): koh-doh
- mano (hand): mah-noh
- dedo (finger): deh-doh
- cadera (hip): kah-deh-rah
- pierna (leg): pyehr-nah
- rodilla (knee): roh-dee-yah
- tobillo (ankle): toh-bee-yoh
- pie (foot): pyeh
- dedo del pie (toe): deh-doh del pyeh

Now that we have some basic vocabulary, let's explore some fun ways to reinforce it. You can create flashcards with images of each body part and the corresponding word in Spanish. Or, you can practice describing body parts using complete sentences. For example, "Tengo ojos verdes" (I have green eyes) or "Me duele la cabeza" (My head hurts).

CLOTHES AND ACCESSORIES

It's time to talk about "ropa" (clothes) and "accesorios" (accesories). Here's a list of some common vocabulary words to get you started:

- la camisa (the shirt): lah kah-mee-sah
- el pantalón (the pants): el pan-tah-lohn
- la falda (the skirt): lah fahl-dah
- el vestido (the dress): el be-stee-doh
- los zapatos (the shoes): lohs sah-pah-tohs
- las botas (the boots): lahs boh-tahs
- las zapatillas (the sneakers): lahs sah-pah-tee-yahs
- los calcetines (the socks): lohs kahl-seh-tee-nehs
- la corbata (the tie): lah kohr-bah-tah
- el sombrero (the hat): el sohm-breh-roh
- la bufanda (the scarf): lah boo-fahn-dah
- los guantes (the gloves): lohs gwahn-tehs
- las gafas (the glasses): lahs gah-fahs
- el reloj (the watch): el reh-loh
- el bolso (the purse): el bohl-soh

You'll notice that this time I included the articles before the words. This is because, in Spanish, nouns and adjectives have gender, contrary to English where they are gender neutral.

When an object is feminine we say "la" (the), and when it is masculine we use "el" (the). While in English you would say "the car" or "the house," in Spanish you would say "el auto" or "la casa."

Don't worry too much about the gender of the objects we learn for now; this is simply so that your brain can build associations between objects and their gender in Spanish.

Now, here's a fun challenge for you: Look at yourself in the mirror and try to name all the clothes and accessories you're wearing in Spanish. Don't worry if you don't know all the words yet, just give it a try! This is a great way to reinforce your vocabulary and get into the habit of using Spanish in your daily life.

FAMILY AND RELATIONSHIPS

Did you know that family is a very important aspect of Spanish culture? The Spanish language has many words to describe different family members, and it's essential to know them if you want to communicate effectively with native speakers.

So, let's start with the list of family members in Spanish:

- abuela (grandmother): ah-bweh-lah
- abuelo (grandfather): ah-bweh-loh
- madre (mother): mah-dreh
- padre (father): pah-dreh
- hijo/hija (son/daughter): ee-hoh/ee-hah
- hermano/hermana (brother/sister): ehr-mah-noh/ehr-mah-nah
- tío/tía (uncle/aunt): tee-oh/tee-ah
- sobrino/sobrina (nephew/niece): soh-bree-noh/soh-bree-nah
- primo/prima (cousin): pree-moh/pree-mah
- esposo/esposa (husband/wife): ehs-poh-soh/ehs-poh-sah

Now, here comes the fun part! Make a list of the names of your own family members. Do not write the words in English next to each family member, but in Spanish. For example, if you have a sister named Mary, you would write "Hermana: Mary." This way, you will begin to link these concepts with your context.

Remember, it's important to put the vocabulary into context by using your own family members' names. This will help you remember the words more easily and make the learning experience more enjoyable.

AROUND THE HOME

Now, let's move on and learn some useful vocabulary for around the home!

Baño (bathroom): bah-nyoh

- la bañera (the bathtub): lah bahn-yeh-rah
- el inodoro (the toilet): el ee-noh-doh-roh
- el lavabo (the sink): el lah-bah-boh
- la ducha (the shower): lah doo-chah
- la toalla (the towel): lah toh-ah-yah
- el jabón (the soap): el hah-bohn

Sala de estar (living room): sah-lah deh ehs-tahr

- el sofá (the sofa): el soh-fah
- la mesa (the table): lah meh-sah
- la televisión (the television): lah teh-lee-bee-syohn
- la silla (the chair): lah see-yah

- la alfombra (the rug): lah ahl-fohm-brah
- el estante (the bookshelf): el ehs-tahn-teh
- el cuadro (the painting): el kooah-droh

Cocina (kitchen): koh-see-nah

- la estufa (the stove): lah ehs-too-fah
- el refrigerador (the refrigerator): el reh-free-heh-rah-dohr
- el horno (the oven): el ohr-noh
- el fregadero (the sink): el freh-gah-deh-roh
- el plato (the plate): el plah-toh
- el tenedor (the fork): el teh-neh-dohr
- el cuchillo (the knife): el koo-chee-yoh
- la cuchara (the spoon): lah koo-chah-rah
- el vaso (the glass): el bah-soh
- la taza (the cup): lah tah-sah

Cuarto (bedroom): kwahr-toh

- la cama (the bed): lah kah-mah
- las sábanas (the sheets): lahs sah-bah-nahs
- el armario (the closet): el ahr-mah-ryo
- el espejo (the mirror): el ehs-peh-hoh
- la lámpara (the lamp): lah lahmpah-rah
- el reloj despertador (the alarm clock): el reh-loh hdehs-pehr-tah-dohr
- la mesita de noche (the nightstand): lah meh-see-tah deh noh-cheh
- la almohada (the pillow): lah al-moh-ah-dah

Jardín (garden): hahr-deen

- el césped (the lawn): el seh-spehd
- la maceta (the pot): lah mah-seh-tah
- el árbol (the tree): el ahr-bohl
- la flor (the flower): lah flohr
- la manguera (the hose): lah mahn-geh-rah
- la pala (the shovel): lah pah-lah

It's time to put it into practice! I challenge you to (roughly) sketch your own home and label the main parts in Spanish. This will help reinforce the vocabulary you just learned and give you a visual representation of the words. Have fun!

TRAVEL AND TRANSPORT

Are you ready to hit the road and explore beautiful Spanish-speaking countries? Then let's start by learning some essential Spanish vocabulary related to travel and transportation!

- Vacaciones (vacations): bah-kah-see-yoh-ness
- el coche/carro/auto (car): el koh-cheh/kah-rroh/ow-toh
- el metro (subway): el meh-troh
- El avión (the plane): ehl ah-vee-ohn
- el aeropuerto (airport): el ah-eh-roh-pwer-toh
- el barco (boat): el bar-koh
- la maleta (suitcase): lah mah-leh-tah
- el billete (ticket): el bee-yeh-teh
- el pasaporte (passport): el pah-sah-pohr-teh
- la carretera (road): lah kah-reh-teh-rah

- la estación (station): lah es-tah-see-yohn
- el equipaje (luggage): el eh-kee-pah-heh

Meet Mary, a travel enthusiast who is going on a holiday to a beautiful island. She will travel by car, metro, and plane to reach her destination.

Mary starts by packing her "maleta" with all the necessary things for her trip, including "ropa," "zapatos," "protector solar," and "gafas de sol." She also makes sure to carry her "billetera" and "pasaporte" with her as they are essential for travel.

Next, she gets into her "coche" and hits the "carretera" towards the city. The road is long and winding, but Mary enjoys the scenic beauty and uses the opportunity to practice her Spanish by singing along to the Spanish radio station.

Once she reaches the city, she parks her car and takes the "metro" to the "aeropuerto." She buys her "billete" and goes through security with her "pasaporte." After some duty-free shopping, she boards the "avión" to the island.

On the "avión," Mary meets some friendly locals and practices her Spanish skills by having a conversation with them. Finally, she reaches the island and collects her "equipaje" before heading to the hotel.

Now, it's your turn! Can you translate all the Spanish vocabulary words Mary used on her journey? Learning new vocabulary is essential for successful travel and a fun way to challenge your brain. So, let's get started and prepare for your next adventure!

Deducing the meaning of words from context is an almost automatic mechanism that leads us to learn a lot when we are exposed to a new language.

JOBS AND THE OFFICE

Enough fun. It's time to talk about work.

Below is a chart with two columns. The first column lists common job titles in Spanish, and the second column is blank for you to try and guess the occupation (many are obvious like "dentista"). But wait! Before you look at the English translations under the chart, try and cover it up and see how many job titles you can guess based on the Spanish word alone.

Spanish Word	Occupation
Cajero	
Abogado	
Cocinero	
Dentista	
Enfermero	
Escritor	

Ingeniero	
Médico	
Periodista	
Programador	
Secretario	
Profesor	

How did you do? Don't worry if you didn't get them all right, that's what we're here to learn! Let's go through the list of jobs in Spanish and their English translations:

- cajero (cashier): kah-heh-roh
- abogado (lawyer): ah-boh-gah-doh
- cocinero (chef): koh-see-neh-roh
- dentista (dentist): den-tee-stah
- enfermero (nurse): ehn-fehr-meh-roh
- escritor (writer): ess-kree-tor
- ingeniero (engineer): een-heh-nee-eh-roh
- médico (doctor): meh-dee-koh
- periodista (journalist): peh-ree-oh-dee-stah
- programador (programmer): proh-grah-mah-dor
- secretario (secretary): seh-kreh-tah-ree-oh
- profesor (teacher): proh-feh-sor
- policia (police officer): poh-lee-see-ah
- vendedor (salesperson): ben-deh-dor

- terapeuta (therapist): teh-rah-pehoo-tah
- dueño de negocios (business owner): doo-eh-nyoh deh neh-goh-see-ohs
- inversionista (investor): een-ver-seeoh-nees-tah
- emprendedor (entrepreneur): em-pren-deh-dor
- deportista (athlete): deh-por-tee-stah
- artista (artist): ar-tees-tah
- científico (scientist): see-en-tee-fee-koh
- político (politician): poh-lee-tee-koh

Now that you have a good base of job titles in Spanish, it's time to reinforce that knowledge. Practice using these words in context by imagining yourself in an office setting or out in the field. You can also try creating flashcards with the Spanish word on one side and the English translation on the other. And don't forget to use these words in conversation with others who speak Spanish. This may be a little embarrassing for you, but it is a fundamental barrier that you have to face. You can read many manuals to learn Spanish, but you won't learn it if you don't speak it.

SCHOOL SUBJECTS

Learning all these words will not only help you communicate better with Spanish-speaking students and teachers, but it will also broaden your knowledge and understanding of the world.

Here are some of the most common school subjects in Spanish:

- matemáticas (mathematics): mah-teh-mah-tee-kahs
- ciencias (science): see-ehn-see-ahs
- historia (history): ees-toh-ree-ah
- geografía (geography): heh-oh-grah-fee-ah
- lengua y literatura (language and literature): lehn-gwah ee lee-teh-rah-too-rah
- arte (art): ahr-teh
- música (music): moo-see-kah
- educación física (physical education): eh-doo-kah-see-ohn fee-see-kah
- tecnología (technology): tehk-noh-loh-hee-ah
- idiomas (languages): ee-dee-oh-mahs

Try to memorize these words by creating associations with them or making flashcards. Practice saying them out loud and using them in sentences to help you remember them better.

Now that you have learned these new words, it's time to practice! Test yourself by trying to write a sentence using each of these school subjects in Spanish. You can also practice listening and comprehension by watching videos in Spanish about these topics —with English subtitles, of course.

DOMESTIC CHORES

Now, let's talk about household chores! It's not the most glamorous topic, but it's certainly an important one. After all, keeping your living space clean and organized can make a big difference in your overall well-being.

So, let's dive into some vocabulary that will help you tackle those domestic duties with ease. Here are some key verbs to keep in mind:

- limpiar (to clean): leem-pyahr
- desempolvar (to dust): dehs-ehm-pohl-bahr
- barrer (to sweep): bah-rehr
- fregar (to mop): freh-gahr
- aspirar (to vacuum): ah-spee-rahr
- lavar (to wash): lah-bahr
- lavar la ropa (to do the laundry): lah-bahr lah roh-pah
- secar (to dry): seh-kahr
- planchar (to iron): plahn-chahr
- colgar (to hang): kohl-gahr
- recoger (to pick up): reh-koh-hehr
- quitar (to remove): kee-tahr
- sacar la basura (to take out the trash): sah-kahr lah bah-soo-rah
- cortar el césped (to mow): kohr-tahr ehl sehsped
- regar (to water): reh-gahr
- clasificar (to sort): klah-see-fee-kahr

With these verbs in your vocabulary arsenal, you'll be able to describe exactly what needs to be done around the house. Whether it's sweeping up the kitchen (barrer la cocina), vacuuming the living room (aspirar la sala de estar), or doing laundry (lavar ropa), you'll be able to communicate your needs clearly.

ANIMALS

Animals come in all shapes and sizes, and Spanish has a rich vocabulary to describe them all. Let's start with popular pets and farm animals:

- perro (dog): peh-roh
- gato (cat): gah-toh
- conejo (rabbit): koh-neh-hoh
- pájaro (bird): pah-hah-roh
- caballo (horse): kah-bah-yoh
- vaca (cow): bah-kah
- cerdo (pig): sehr-doh
- oveja (sheep): oh-veh-hah
- gallina (chicken): gah-yee-nah
- pato (duck): pah-toh

Moving on to land animals:

- león (lion): leh-ohn
- tigre (tiger): tee-greh
- mono (monkey): moh-noh
- elefante (elephant): eh-leh-fahn-teh
- jirafa (giraffe): hee-rah-fah

- zorro (fox): soh-roh
- oso (bear): oh-soh
- lobo (wolf): loh-boh
- cebra (zebra): seh-brah
- rinoceronte (rhinoceros): ree-noh-seh-rohn-teh

And lastly, aquatic animals:

- tiburón (shark): tee-boo-rohn
- ballena (whale): bah-yeh-nah
- delfín (dolphin): dehl-feen
- pulpo (octopus): pool-poh
- caballito de mar (seahorse): kah-bah-yee-toh deh mahr
- pez (fish): pehz
- cangrejo (crab): kahn-greh-hoh
- langosta (lobster): lahng-goh-stah
- medusa (jellyfish): meh-doo-sah
- estrella de mar (starfish): ehs-treh-yah deh mahr

HOBBIES

Now that we have explored the world of animals, let's shift gears and delve into the realm of personal interests and hobbies. Just as the animal kingdom boasts a remarkable array of species, humans, too, exhibit a vast range of passions and activities that captivate their hearts and minds. So, let's learn some of the most common hobbies and interests in Spanish:

- bailar (to dance): bah-ee-lahr
- cocinar (to cook): koh-see-nahr

- leer (to read): leh-ehr
- ver películas (to watch movies): behr peh-lee-koo-lahs
- escuchar música (to listen to music): ehs-koo-char moo-see-kah
- jugar videojuegos (to play video games): hoo-gahr bee-deh-oh-hweh-gohs
- hacer deporte (to do sports): ah-sehr deh-pohr-teh
- pintar (to paint): peen-tahr
- viajar (to travel): bee-ah-hahr
- escribir (to write): ehs-kree-beer

To practice talking about your hobbies, try using the phrase "Me gusta (meh goos-tah)" which means "I like." For example, "Me gusta bailar (meh goos-tah bahy-lahr)" means "I like dancing." You can also use "No me gusta (noh meh goos-tah)," which means "I don't like."

You now have a diverse range of vocabulary under your belt. By learning about animals, jobs, and hobbies, you've opened up a world of possibilities in your Spanish-speaking journey. From discussing your pets and favorite animals to talking about your job and hobbies, you'll have plenty to say in conversations with native Spanish speakers. But don't stop here! In the next chapter, we'll dive deeper into time expressions, so you can add more context and meaning to your newfound vocabulary. Keep up the good work!

PRACTICE AND VOCABULARY

1. **Label everything!** You can label different elements according to their color and shape. You can also stick a list on the door of your closet with the name of each item of clothing and, just in case, a drawing or two.
2. **Play the role**: Your family and pets may not like that you label them so instead try to always refer to them with the word in Spanish. For example, you can have your mom on your cell phone as "mamá" instead of "mom."
3. **Practice "I like" and "I don't like"**: You can build many sentences from what you know so far. List the animals, clothes, things, and jobs you like, as well as those you don't. For example: "I like the lion" or "I don't like to work."
4. **Read the text and answer the questions below. Try not to check the translation unless is necessary.**

Lola es una niña pequeña. Ella tiene una bufanda roja y unas zapatillas amarillas. Hoy se siente aventurera y decide salir al parque. Allí ve muchas cosas de colores diferentes, como una flor naranja, un elefante gris, un cangrejo rojo y una estrella de mar morada. También ve a un deportista corriendo y a un policía patrullando en su coche.

Luego de jugar un rato, Lola regresa a casa y ayuda a su abuela a fregar los platos y a sacar la basura. Después de lavar sus manos, Lola se sienta en el sofá y lee una historia sobre un conejo que vive en el bosque. Mientras lee, se rasca la espalda. Está molesta porque le duele un poco la rodilla y el pie. Finalmente, Lola se queda dormida.

Translation:

Lola is a little girl. She has a red scarf and yellow sneakers. Today, she feels adventurous and decides to go out to the park. There she sees many things of different colors, such as an orange flower, a gray elephant, a red crab, and a purple starfish. She also sees a jogging athlete and a patrolling police officer in her car.

After playing for a while, Lola returns home and helps her grandmother wash the dishes and take out the trash. After washing her hands, Lola sits on the sofa and reads a story about a rabbit that lives in the forest. As she reads, she scratches her back. She is upset because her knee and foot hurt a little. Finally, Lola falls asleep.

Questions:

1. ¿Cómo se llama la niña de la historia?
2. ¿De qué color es la bufanda de Lola?
3. ¿Qué animal de color rojo ve Lola en el parque?
4. ¿Qué hace Lola cuando regresa a casa?
5. ¿Por qué está molesta Lola mientras lee la historia?

Answers:

1. Lola. (Lola.)
2. Roja. (Red.)
3. Un cangrejo. (A crab.)

4. Ayuda a su abuela a fregar los platos y a sacar la basura. (She helps her grandmother wash the dishes and take out the garbage.)

5. Porque le duele un poco la rodilla y el pie. (Because her knee and foot hurt a little.)

NUMBERS AND TIME

In this chapter, we will cover the essentials of numbers and time in Spanish. We'll start with the basics, such as cardinal and ordinal numbers, and progress to more complex expressions like dates and telling time, and talking about the weather.

Along the way, I'll provide useful tips and tricks to make sure you're confident in using these expressions in real-life situations. By the end of this chapter, you'll be able to express dates and times accurately and avoid any embarrassing or costly misunderstandings. So, let's dive in and get started with the world of Spanish numbers and time!

CARDINAL AND ORDINAL NUMBERS

Let's start with cardinal numbers, which are used to count things or people.

Here are the first 20 cardinal numbers:

0. cero (ceh-roh)
1. uno (oo-noh)
2. dos (dohs)
3. tres (trehs)
4. cuatro (kwat-roh)
5. cinco (seen-koh)
6. seis (sayss)
7. siete (syeh-teh)
8. ocho (oh-choh)
9. nueve (nweh-veh)
10. diez (dyehs)
11. once (ohn-seh)
12. doce (doh-seh)
13. trece (treh-seh)
14. catorce (kah-tor-seh)
15. quince (keen-seh)
16. dieciséis (dyeh-see-sees)
17. diecisiete (dyeh-see-syeh-teh)
18. dieciocho (dyeh-see-oh-choh)
19. diecinueve (dyeh-see-nweh-veh)
20. veinte (beyn-teh)

In Spanish, numbers are composed by using the same system as in English with the exception of the numbers 11 through 15. In English, these numbers are composed of a "teen" suffix (thirteen, fourteen, fifteen), but in Spanish, they are formed by adding the suffix -ce to the corresponding root number. For example, eleven in Spanish is "once" (1 + 10), and twelve is "doce" (2 + 10).

After 15, the root number is used followed by the conjunction "y" (and) and the corresponding unit number. For example, 16 is "dieciséis" (10 + 6), 17 is "diecisiete" (10 + 7), and so on.

Here you have some examples of numbers above 20:

- 24: veinticuatro (vayn-tee-kwah-troh)
- 31: treinta y uno (trayn-tah ee oo-noh)
- 46: cuarenta y seis (kwar-en-tah ee seis)
- 58: cincuenta y ocho (seen-kwen-tah ee oh-choh)
- 60: sesenta (seh-sehn-tah)
- 79: setenta y nueve (seh-ten-tah ee noo-eh-veh)
- 82: ochenta y dos (oh-chen-tah ee dohs)
- 95: noventa y cinco (noh-ven-tah ee seen-koh)
- 100: cien (syehn)
- 120: ciento veinte (see-ehn-toh vayn-teh)

Additionally, when expressing numbers in Spanish, it's common to use a period instead of a comma to separate the decimal and whole numbers. For example, the number 3.14 in Spanish would be written as 3,14, since the dot is used to separate magnitude orders—in Spanish, you would write 1.000.000 for a million, while in English you would write 1,000,000. In short, where dots are used in English, commas are used in Spanish and vice versa.

Here you have some examples to see it more clearly:

- 2.5 (English) - 2,5 (Spanish)
- 3,567.89 (English) - 3.567,89 (Spanish)
- 12,345,678 (English) - 12.345.678 (Spanish)
- 0.75 (English) - 0,75 (Spanish)

Now, let's move on to the ordinal numbers, which are used to indicate the position of something in a series. Here are the first 10 ordinal numbers:

1. primero (pree-meh-roh): first
2. segundo (seh-goon-doh): second
3. tercero (tehr-seh-roh): third
4. cuarto (kwar-toh): fourth
5. quinto (keen-toh): fifth
6. sexto (seks-toh): sixth
7. séptimo (sep-tee-moh): seventh
8. octavo (ohk-tah-voh): eighth
9. noveno (noh-beh-noh): ninth
10. décimo (deh-see-moh): tenth

Knowing how to say numbers up to the thousands can also come in handy.

Here's a brief guide on how to say larger numbers in Spanish:

- 1.000: mil (meel)
- 10.000: diez mil (dyehss meel)
- 100.000: cien mil (syehn meel)

- 1.000.000: un millón (oon mee-yohn)

TELLING THE TIME

When it comes to telling time, the 24-hour clock is commonly used in Spain. So, for example, 3:00 pm would be expressed as "15:00." However, it's also common to use the 12-hour clock in everyday conversation. To say "in the morning" or "in the after-noon/evening," use the phrases "de la mañana" or "de la tarde/noche," respectively.

As we all know, time is of the essence, and mastering this skill will help you avoid unnecessary confusion and embarrassment.

Let's start with the basics, shall we? To say "It's 1 o'clock" in Spanish, you simply say "Es la una." Easy peasy, right? But after that, things get a little trickier.

For all the other hours, you'll need to use "son las" followed by the number. For example, "Son las dos" means "It's 2 o'clock." And if you want to say "It's half past 2," you would say "Son las dos y media."

Moving on to the minutes, you can use the phrase "y" to indicate "and." For example, "Son las tres y quince" means "It's 3:15." You can also use the phrase "menos" to indicate "minus." So "Son las cuatro menos veinte" means "It's 3:40."

It may seem daunting at first, but with practice, you'll soon be telling time like a pro! To help you on your journey, here are some examples of how to tell the time in Spanish:

- Es la una (es lah oo-nah): It's one o'clock
- Son las dos (sohn lahs dohs): It's two o'clock
- Son las tres y cuarto (sohn lahs trayz ee kwahr-toh): It's quarter past three
- Son las cuatro y media (sohn lahs kwah-troh ee mah-dee-ah): It's half past four
- Son las cinco y cuarenta y cinco (sohn lahs seen-koh ee kwah-rehn-tah ee seen-koh): It's five forty-five.
- Son las seis en punto (sohn lahs sayz ehn poon-toh): It's six o'clock sharp
- Son las siete y diez (sohn lahs syeh-teh ee dyehs): It's ten past seven
- Son las ocho y veinte (sohn lahs oh-choh ee beyn-teh): It's twenty past eight
- Son las nueve y media (sohn lahs nweh-veh ee meh-dyah): It's half past nine
- Son las diez menos veinticinco (sohn lahs dyehs meh-nohs beyn-tee-seen-koh): It's twenty-five to ten

DAYS, MONTHS, AND SEASONS

Now, it's time to cover days, months, and seasons.

Let's start with the days of the week:

- Lunes (loo-nehs): Monday
- Martes (mahr-tehs): Tuesday
- Miércoles (mee-ehr-koh-lehs): Wednesday
- Jueves (hweh-behs): Thursday
- Viernes (bee-ehr-nehs): Friday

- Sábado (sah-bah-doh): Saturday
- Domingo (doh-meen-goh): Sunday

Now, let's move on to the months of the year:

- Enero (eh-neh-roh): January
- Febrero (feh-breh-roh): February
- Marzo (mahr-soh): March
- Abril (ah-breehl): April
- Mayo (mah-yoh): May
- Junio (hoo-nee-oh): June
- Julio (hoo-lee-oh): July
- Agosto (ah-goh-stoh): August
- Septiembre (sehp-tee-yehm-breh): September
- Octubre (ohk-too-breh): October
- Noviembre (noh-byehm-breh): November
- Diciembre (dee-see-yehm-breh): December

It's also important to know the seasons in Spanish:

- Primavera (pree-mah-veh-rah): Spring
- Verano (beh-rah-noh): Summer
- Otoño (oh-toh-nyoh): Fall
- Invierno (een-vyehr-noh): Winter

When discussing a date, it's essential to note that Spanish uses cardinal numbers rather than ordinal numbers, which are used in English. For example, in English, we say "March 15th," while in Spanish, it is "15 de marzo." Additionally, years in Spanish are said as complete numbers. For example, the year 2023 is "dos mil veintitrés," unlike English, where you would split the year into two parts (twenty-twenty-three for 2023).

TALKING ABOUT THE WEATHER

When it comes to discussing the weather in Spanish, it's important to know how to express the temperature, as well as other conditions like rain, snow, wind, and humidity. Here are some common weather expressions in Spanish:

- Está frío (eh-stah free-oh): It's cold.
- Está caluroso (eh-stah kah-loo-rho-soh): It's hot.
- Está nevado (eh-stah neh-vah-doh): It's snowy.
- Está lluvioso (eh-stah yoo-vee-oh-soh): It's rainy.
- Está ventoso (eh-stah ben-toh-soh): It's windy.
- Está húmedo (eh-stah oo-meh-doh): It's humid.

It's important to note that these expressions use the verb "estar" (to be) instead of "ser" (to be) because weather conditions are temporary and subject to change.

When describing temperature, you will have to use the Celsius scale, since all Spanish-speaking countries use the International Metric System units. In Spanish, Celsius is usually used, and it's expressed as "grados Celsius" or just "grados" for short.

For example:

- Hace veinte grados Celsius: It's 20 degrees Celsius. (ah-seh beyn-teh grah-dohs sehl-see-yoos)

- Hace treinta y dos grados: It's 32 degrees. (ah-seh trehn-tah ee dohs grah-dohs)

By learning these expressions, you'll be able to discuss the weather and make small talk with others. Plus, you'll be able to understand weather forecasts and plan your activities accordingly.

ADVERBS OF TIME

Adverbs of time are essential in Spanish to express when an action occurred or how frequently it happens. Here is a list of some common adverbs of time that you can use in your everyday conversations:

- ahora (ah-oh-rah): now
- antes (ahn-tes): before
- después (dehs-pwehs): after
- pronto (prohn-toh): soon
- tarde (tar-deh): late
- temprano (tem-pran-oh): early
- nunca (noon-kah): never
- siempre (see-ehm-preh): always

Additionally, here are some time expressions that can be helpful to communicate more specific points in time:

- hoy (oi): today
- ayer (ah-yehr): yesterday
- mañana (mah-nyah-nah): tomorrow

- la semana pasada (lah se-man-ah pah-sa-dah): last week
- el mes pasado (el mes pah-sa-doh): last month
- el año pasado (el ahn-yo pah-sa-doh): last year
- la próxima semana (lah proh-ksih-mah se-man-ah): next week
- el próximo mes (el proh-ksih-moh mes): next month
- el próximo año (el proh-ksih-moh ahn-yo): next year
- mañana (mah-nyah-nah): morning
- mediodía (meh-dee-oh-dee-ah): noon
- tarde (tahr-deh): afternoon
- noche (noh-cheh): night
- madrugada (mah-droo-gah-dah): early morning/dawn

With these adverbs and expressions of time, you'll be able to confidently communicate when certain things happen and for how long.

PRACTICE AND VOCABULARY

1. In order to help you practice your skills in using numbers and time expressions, I have prepared a list of 25 phrases for you to translate. Make sure to write your translations to Spanish in the space provided after the phrase:

A. 5:25 am on Monday: _____

B. Monday the 16th of June: _____

C. May 1853: _____

D. The day before yesterday: _____

E. 3:45 pm: _____

F. September 12th, 2005: _____

G. In two weeks: _____

H. Quarter past nine: _____

I. Next Thursday at 8 am: _____

J. December 31st, 1999: _____

K. Five minutes to eleven: _____

L. 13:50 hours: _____

M. Friday the 13th: _____

N. Last Friday: _____

O. August 1st, 2022: _____

P. 11:11 pm: _____

Q. Second Monday in January: _____

R. Three days ago: _____

S. October 23rd, 1976: _____

T. Half past six: _____

U. At noon: _____

V. First week of the month: _____

W. At early morning: _____

X. April 15th, 2024: _____

Y. Half past nine in the evening: _____

Answers:

A. 5:25 de la madrugada del lunes

B. Lunes 16 de junio

C. Mayo de 1853

D. Anteayer

E. 3:45 de la tarde

F. 12 de septiembre de 2005

G. En dos semanas

H. Las nueve y cuarto

I. El próximo jueves a las 8 de la mañana

J. 31 de diciembre de 1999

K. Faltan cinco minutos para las once

L. 13:50 horas

M. Viernes 13

N. El viernes pasado

O. 1 de agosto de 2022

P. 11:11 de la noche

Q. Segundo lunes de enero

R. Hace tres días

S. 23 de octubre de 1976

T. Las seis y media

U. Al mediodía

V. La primera semana del mes

W. A primera hora de la mañana

X. 15 de abril de 2024

Y. Las nueve y media de la noche

2. Read and answer:

Es un día caluroso de verano en septiembre. Son las tres y cuarto de la tarde y hace treinta y dos grados. En este momento, estoy sentado en la oficina, tratando de concentrarme en mi trabajo. Ayer fue un día muy ocupado, pero hoy parece que será un poco más tranquilo.

El próximo mes, estaré de vacaciones. Me iré a una playa hermosa en México y estoy muy emocionado. Esta noche, voy a hacer planes para mi viaje y pensar en todo lo que quiero hacer. Primero, quiero disfrutar de la playa y el mar. Segundo, quiero visitar algunas ruinas antiguas. Y tercero, quiero probar la comida local. Me encanta la comida mexicana. Creo que diez mil pesos serán suficientes para cubrir todos mis gastos durante el viaje.

Translation:

It is a hot summer day in September. It's a quarter past three in the afternoon and it's thirty-two degrees. Right now, I'm sitting in the office, trying to focus on my work. Yesterday was a very busy day, but today it looks like it will be a bit calmer.

Next month, I'll be on vacation. I'm going to a beautiful beach in Mexico and I'm very excited. Tonight, I'm going to make plans for my trip and think about everything I want to do. First, I want to enjoy the beach and the sea. Second, I want to visit some ancient ruins. And third, I want to try the local food. I love Mexican food. I think that ten thousand pesos will be enough to cover all my expenses during the trip.

Questions:

1. ¿En qué mes está ambientada la historia?
2. ¿Dónde irá de vacaciones el narrador?
3. ¿Qué quiere hacer el narrador durante su viaje?
4. ¿Cuánto dinero piensa que será suficiente para su viaje?

Answers:

1. La historia está ambientada en septiembre. (The story is set in September.)
2. El narrador irá de vacaciones a una playa hermosa en México. (The narrator will go on vacation to a beautiful beach in Mexico.)
3. El narrador quiere disfrutar de la playa y el mar, visitar algunas ruinas antiguas y probar la comida local. (The narrator wants to enjoy the beach and sea, visit some ancient ruins, and try the local food.)
4. El narrador piensa que diez mil pesos serán suficientes para cubrir todos sus gastos durante el viaje. (The narrator thinks that ten thousand pesos will be enough to cover all his expenses during the trip.)

Don't worry if you find some of these phrases challenging at first. Remember to take your time and use your knowledge of the vocabulary and grammar that we've covered in this chapter. With a little practice, you'll be able to recognize dates and times easily and use them effectively in your everyday communication.

You can use this list as a reference tool as you continue to develop your language skills. Good luck!

4

COMMON WORDS AND PHRASES
FOR EVERYDAY SITUATIONS

Welcome to Chapter 4 of our Spanish language learning journey! By this point, you've learned essential vocabulary and gained some insights into the rich history of the language. Now, it's time to focus on everyday conversations and build your confidence in speaking Spanish.

In this chapter, we'll be covering common words and phrases that you can use in a wide range of situations. But more than that, I'll also give you the tools to maintain and deepen your conversations by asking questions and exploring topics in more detail.

Meet Sarah, a curious and open-minded traveler who has always been fascinated by Spanish culture. She was on a backpacking trip through Spain and stumbled upon a small village that piqued her interest. As she explored the village, she noticed something peculiar: the locals seemed to greet each other with various greetings, but there didn't seem to be any particular rule on when to use which one.

She would hear "Hola" or "Buenos días" in the morning, "Adiós" or "Hasta luego" in the evening, and "Hasta mañana" or "Hasta pronto" throughout the day. Sarah found this confusing, and she couldn't help but wonder if she was doing something wrong by not following the proper protocol.

To make matters worse, she discovered that the rules for time were also different from what she was used to. In English, it's customary to say "Good morning" until noon, "Good afternoon" from noon until evening, and "Good evening" from evening until night. However, in this village, people would say "Buenas tardes" (good afternoon) after they had eaten lunch, which could be as early as 11:30 am.

This only added to Sarah's confusion, as she struggled to adapt to the unfamiliar cultural norms. She would often find herself second-guessing which greeting to use or when to use it. Despite this, Sarah appreciated the warm and welcoming nature of the locals and continued to explore the village with an open mind, eager to learn more about their unique way of life.

If you are like Sarah, you're probably a little confused too about the different greetings that Spanish speakers use, but don't worry! By the end of this chapter, you'll have a good grasp on these cultural nuances and the confidence to navigate everyday conversations with ease, as Sarah did.

FIRST IMPRESSIONS

Here you have a list with useful examples for diverse situations:

Saludos (Greetings):

- ¡Hola! (oh-lah): Hello!
- ¡Buenos días! (bweh-nohs dee-as): Good morning!
- ¡Buenas tardes! (bweh-nahs tar-des): Good afternoon!
- ¡Buenas noches! (bweh-nahs noh-ches): Good evening/night!
- ¡Hola, qué tal? (oh-lah, keh tal): Hi, how are you?
- ¿Cómo estás? (koh-moh ehs-tahs): How are you?
- ¿Qué pasa? (keh pah-sah): What's up?
- ¡Encantado/a! (en-kahn-tah-doh/dah): Nice to meet you!
- ¡Mucho gusto! (moo-choh goos-toh): Nice to meet you!
- ¡Bienvenido/a! (bee-en-veh-nee-doh/dah): Welcome!
- ¡Saludos! (sah-lu-dohs): Greetings!

Presentaciones (Introductions):

- Me llamo [name]. (meh yah-moh): My name is [name].
- Soy de [place]. (soy deh): I'm from [place].
- ¿Y tú? (ee too): And you?
- Él/Ella es [name]. (el/eh-yah es): He/She is [name].
- Éstos son mis amigos. (ehs-tohs sohn mees ah-mee-gohs): These are my friends.
- Permíteme presentarte a... (pehr-mee-teh-meh preh-sen-tar-teh ah): Allow me to introduce you to...

Despedidas (Farewells):

- ¡Adiós! (ah-dee-ohs): Goodbye!
- ¡Hasta luego! (ahs-tah loo-eh-goh): See you later!
- ¡Hasta pronto! (ahs-tah prohn-toh): See you soon!
- ¡Nos vemos! (nohs veh-mohs): See you!
- ¡Chao! (chow): Bye!
- ¡Que tengas un buen día! (keh tehn-gahs un bwehn dee-ah): Have a nice day!
- ¡Que descanses! (keh dehs-kahn-sehs: Rest well!
- ¡Hasta la próxima! (ahs-tah lah proks-ee-mah): Until next time!

Saludos de festividades (Holiday Greetings):

- ¡Feliz Navidad! (feh-lees nah-vee-dahd): Merry Christmas!
- ¡Feliz Año Nuevo! (feh-lees ahn-yoh new-eh-voh): Happy New Year!
- ¡Felices Fiestas! (feh-lee-sehs fyehs-tahs): Happy Holidays!
- ¡Feliz Día de Acción de Gracias! (feh-lees dee-ah deh ahk-see-on deh grah-see-ahs): Happy Thanksgiving!
- ¡Feliz Día de San Valentín! (feh-lees dee-ah deh sahn bah-lehn-teen): Happy Valentine's Day!
- ¡Felíz día de los Muertos! (feh-lees dee-ah deh lohs mwehr-tohs): Happy Day of the Dead!
- ¡Feliz Día de la Madre! (feh-lees dee-ah deh lah mah-dreh): Happy Mother's Day!

- ¡Feliz Día del Padre! (feh-lees dee-ah del pah-dreh): Happy Father's Day!
- ¡Feliz cumpleaños! (feh-lees koom-ple-ah-nyohs): Happy Birthday!

Have you ever been in a conversation with someone and wanted to ask a question but didn't know how? Or maybe you were asked a question in Spanish but had no idea what was being asked? Now, we will cover the eight question words in Spanish and how to use them. Plus, we will also explore how to ask and answer both closed and open-ended questions. By the end, you'll be able to confidently participate in any conversation!

ASKING AND ANSWERING QUESTIONS

First, let's take a look at the eight question words in Spanish:

- ¿Quién? (khi-ehn): Who?
- ¿Qué? (keh): What?
- ¿Cuál? (kwahl): Which?
- ¿Dónde? (dohn-deh): Where?
- ¿Cuándo? (kwahn-doh): When?
- ¿Por qué? (pohr-keh): Why?
- ¿Cómo? (koh-moh): How?
- ¿Cuánto/a? (kwahn-toh/ah): How much/many?

Remember to pay attention to the accents on question words. Without an accent, it's a relative pronoun. And in written Spanish, there is an upside-down question mark at the beginning of the sentence. This is because there are no auxiliary verbs to indicate that the sentence is a question. In Spanish, you write a question the same as a statement. Except for the accent marks, question marks, and the tonality with which the phrase is said, both are indistinguishable. That is why it is important to pay attention to these details. For example, the question "¿Hoy está frío?" (Is it cold today?) is very similar to the statement "Hoy está frío" (Today is cold).

Closed questions are those that require a yes or no answer. Here are some examples:

- ¿Eres de España? (eh-res deh eh-span-ya): Are you from Spain?
- ¿Hablas español? (ah-blahs eh-spah-nyol): Do you speak Spanish?
- ¿Te gusta la música? (teh goos-ta lah moo-see-kah): Do you like music?
- ¿Has viajado al extranjero? (ahs bee-ah-hah-doh ahl ex-trahn-heh-roh): Have you traveled abroad?
- ¿Estás cansado/a? (ehs-tahs kan-sah-doh/kan-sah-dah): Are you tired?
- ¿Tienes hermanos? (tee-eh-nehs ehr-mah-nohs): Do you have siblings?

Open-ended questions require a more detailed response and cannot be answered with a simple yes or no. Here are some examples:

- ¿Quién eres? (khi-ehn eh-rehs): Who are you?
- ¿Cuándo es tu cumpleaños? (kwan-doh ehs too koom-pleh-ahn-yohs): When is your birthday?
- ¿De dónde eres? (deh dohn-deh eh-rehs): Where are you from?
- ¿Qué tiempo hace hoy? (keh tee-ehm-poh ah-seh oh-ee): What's the weather like today?
- ¿Qué hora es? (keh oh-rah ehs): What time is it?
- ¿Cómo te llamas? (koh-moh teh yah-mahs): What's your name?
- ¿Qué estás haciendo? (keh ehs-tahs ah-see-ehn-doh): What are you doing?
- ¿Cuántos años tienes? (kwahn-tohs ahn-yohs tee-eh-nehs): How old are you?
- ¿Dónde vives? (dohn-deh vee-vehs): Where do you live?
- ¿Qué te gusta hacer en tu tiempo libre? (keh teh goos-ta ah-sehr ehn too tee-ehm-poh lee-breh): What do you like to do in your free time?
- ¿Qué tipo de música te gusta? (keh tee-poh deh moo-see-kah teh goos-ta): What kind of music do you like?
- ¿A qué hora te despiertas normalmente? (ah keh oh-rah teh dehs-pyehr-tahs nohr-mahl-mehn-teh): What time do you usually wake up?

ORDERING FOOD AND DRINKS

Food plays a vital role in the cultures of Spanish-speaking countries, where culinary traditions have been shaped by a rich history and diverse geography. From the spicy flavors of Mexico to the delicate seafood dishes of Spain, each country offers a unique gastronomic experience that is not to be missed. Whether you are exploring the bustling streets of Buenos Aires or the charming plazas of Lima, trying the local cuisine is a must-do activity that will allow you to fully immerse yourself in the culture. To help you navigate the menus and order like a local, here are some common phrases and vocabulary words that you can use when dining at a restaurant:

- ¿Nos puede dar la carta, por favor? (nohs pweh-deh dar lah kahr-tah, pohr fah-bor): Can you give us the menu, please?
- Queremos pedir ahora. (keh-reh-mohs peh-deer aho-rah): We want to order now.
- ¿Cuál es la especialidad de la casa? (kwahl ehs lah ess-peh-see-ahl-ee-dahd deh lah kah-sah): What is the specialty of the house?
- ¿Cuál es la sopa del día? (kwahl ehs lah soh-pah del dee-ah): What is the soup of the day?
- ¿Qué recomienda? (keh reh-koh-mee-ehn-dah): What do you recommend?
- ¿Qué lleva este plato? (keh yeh-bah eh-steh plah-toh): What does this dish have?
- ¿Hay algo sin gluten? (ay ahl-goh seen gloo-ten): Is there anything gluten-free?

- La cuenta, por favor. (lah kwehn-tah, pohr fah-bor): The bill, please.

Here you'll find some useful vocabulary:

- El menú (ehl meh-noo): The menu
- La carta (lah kahr-tah): The menu
- La comida (lah koh-mee-dah): The food
- El plato (ehl plah-toh): The dish
- La sopa (lah soh-pah): The soup
- El arroz (ehl ah-rrohz): The rice
- El pollo (ehl poh-yoh): The chicken
- El pescado (ehl peh-skah-doh): The fish
- El postre (ehl pohs-treh): The dessert
- La cuenta (lah kwehn-tah): The bill

Remember to use "por favor" (please) and "gracias" (thank you) when speaking with the waiter or waitress. Buen provecho! (Enjoy your meal!)

Food and drink vocabulary:

Especias/Condimentos	Spices/Seasonings
Sal	Salt
Pimienta	Pepper
Comino	Cumin
Orégano	Oregano
Tomillo	Thyme
Canela	Cinnamon
Clavo de olor	Clove
Verduras	**Vegetables**
Ajo	Garlic
Cebolla	Onion
Lechuga	Lettuce
Tomate	Tomato
Espinaca	Spinach
Zanahoria	Carrot

Pimiento	Bell pepper
Calabacín/Zapallito	Zucchini
Maiz	Corn
Frutas	**Fruits**
Fresa	Strawberry
Kiwi	Kiwi
Piña	Pineapple
Manzana	Apple
Naranja	Orange
Uva	Grape
Plátano/Banana	Banana
Limón	Lemon
Aguacate	Avocado
Pan	**Bread**
Harina	Flour
Avena	Oats
Cebada	Barley
Granos	**Grains**
Arroz	Rice
Quinoa	Quinoa

Carnes	Meats
Carne de res	Beef
Cerdo	Pork
Mariscos	Seafood
Bebidas	**Drinks**
Agua	Water
Té	Tea
Café	Coffee
Refresco/Gaseosa	Soft drink/Soda
Cerveza	Beer
Vino	Wine

Here's a chart with some famous meals from different Spanish-speaking countries and their ingredients:

Dish	Country	Ingredients
Paella	Spain	Arroz (rice), pollo (chicken), conejo (rabbit), mariscos (seafood), pimiento (bell pepper), cebolla (onion), ajo (garlic), tomate (tomato), azafrán (saffron), aceite de oliva (olive oil)
Empanadas	Argentina	Carne (beef), cebolla (onion), pimiento (bell pepper), aceitunas (olives), huevo (egg), aceite (oil), harina (flour), sal (salt)
Ceviche	Peru	Pescado (fish), cebolla (onion), ají (chili), limón (lime), cilantro (coriander), choclo (corn), camote (sweet potato)
Tacos al pastor	Mexico	Carne de cerdo (pork), piña (pineapple), cebolla (onion), cilantro (coriander), limón (lime), tortillas de maíz (corn tortillas)
Gallo pinto	Costa Rica	Arroz (rice), frijoles (beans), cebolla (onion), pimiento (bell pepper), ajo (garlic), cilantro (coriander), sal (salt)
Lomo saltado	Peru	Carne de res (beef), cebolla (onion), tomate (tomato), ajo (garlic), pimiento (bell pepper), papas fritas (French fries), arroz (rice), salsa de soja (soy sauce)
Pabellón criollo	Venezuela	Carne mechada (shredded beef), arroz (rice), frijoles negros (black beans), plátano maduro (ripe plantain), queso blanco (white cheese)

Dish	Country	Ingredients
Arroz con pollo	Puerto Rico	Arroz (rice), pollo (chicken), sofrito (sauce made with onion, garlic, bell pepper, cilantro), ajo (garlic), guisantes (peas), pimiento (bell pepper), caldo de pollo (chicken broth)
Asado	Argentina	Carne de vaca (beef), chorizo (sausage), morcilla (blood sausage), chinchulines (chitterlings), mollejas (sweetbreads), ensalada (salad)

MAKING RESERVATIONS AND APPOINTMENTS

Making reservations and appointments can be a nerve-racking experience when you're trying to do it in a foreign language. But with a little bit of practice and the right vocabulary, you'll be able to schedule meetings, appointments, and reservations with comfort in Spanish.

Here are some essential vocabulary words and phrases to help you navigate through the process:

- Reservar (reh-ser-vahr): to reserve
- Hacer una cita (ah-sehr oo-nah see-tah): to make an appointment
- Confirmar (kohn-feer-mahr): to confirm
- Cancelar (kahn-seh-lahr): to cancel
- Disculpar (dees-kool-pahr): to apologize

When making appointments or reservations, it's important to be clear and concise. Here are some useful phrases to keep in mind:

- ¿Podría reservar una mesa para dos, por favor? (Could I reserve a table for two, please?)
- Quisiera hacer una cita con el doctor. (I would like to make an appointment with the doctor.)
- ¿Podría confirmar mi reserva? (Could you confirm my reservation?)
- Lamentablemente, tengo que cancelar mi cita. (Unfortunately, I have to cancel my appointment.)
- Le pido disculpas por cualquier inconveniente que esto pueda causar. (I apologize for any inconvenience this may cause.)

If you're making appointments or reservations for a business meeting or event, it's important to use formal language. Here are some phrases to help you sound professional:

- Me comunico con usted en relación a... (I am contacting you in regards to...)
- Por medio de la presente, quisiera solicitar una cita con... (I would like to request an appointment with...)
- Por favor, háganme saber si esto es posible. (Please let me know if this is possible.)
- Agradezco de antemano su atención. (I appreciate your attention in advance.)

MONEY MATTERS

It's time to move on to practical vocabulary that can help you navigate your day-to-day life, specifically when it comes to money. Here are some important money-related words and phrases in Spanish that you should know:

- Dinero (dee-neh-roh): Money
- Billete (bee-yeh-teh): Bill
- Moneda (moh-neh-dah): Coin
- Efectivo (eh-fehk-tee-voh): Cash
- Tarjeta de crédito (tahr-heh-tah deh kreh-dee-toh): Credit card
- Cajero automático (kah-heh-roh ow-toh-mah-tee-koh): ATM
- Cambio (kahm-bee-oh): Change
- Precio (preh-see-oh): Price
- Descuento (dehs-kwehn-toh): Discount
- Factura (fahk-too-rah): Invoice
- Recibo (reh-see-boh): Receipt

Now, let's dive into some money-related verbs and phrases:

- Pagar (pah-gahr): To pay
- Cobrar (koh-brahr): To charge or to collect payment
- Comprar (kohm-prahr): To buy
- Vender (benn-dehr): To sell
- Costar (kohs-tahr): To cost
- Ahorrar (ah-oh-hahr): To save
- Gastar (gah-stahr): To spend
- Pedir prestado (peh-deer prehs-tah-doh): To borrow
- Prestar (preh-stahr): To lend
- Devolver (deh-bohl-behr): To return (as in returning borrowed money)

And here are some additional money-related phrases that may come in handy:

- ¿Cuánto cuesta?: How much does it cost?
- Tengo suficiente dinero: I have enough money
- ¿Aceptan tarjeta de crédito?: Do you accept credit card?
- ¿Dónde está el cajero automático más cercano?: Where is the nearest ATM?
- ¿Puedo pagar con dólares/euros?: Can I pay with dollars/euros?
- Quiero cambiar dólares/euros a pesos: I want to exchange dollars/euros for pesos
- No me alcanza: I can't afford (something)
- Está en oferta: It's on sale
- No aceptamos devoluciones: We don't accept returns

Remember, talking about money may vary depending on the country or region you are in. Nevertheless, these phrases should provide you with a good foundation, but don't be afraid to ask for clarification if you are unsure! Again, Spanish speakers love when foreign people are curious about their language.

PUNCTUATION SYMBOLS FOR EMAIL ADDRESSES

You may also be confused about some of the symbols that appear in email addresses. Here's a quick guide to help you out!

- Arroba: "@" at sign
- Punto: "." period
- Guion: "-" hyphen

- Guión bajo: "_" underscore

In Spanish, the at sign is called "arroba," which is derived from the Arabic word for "quarter." It's used in email addresses to separate the user name from the domain name.

The period, or "punto" in Spanish, is used to separate different parts of the domain name.

The hyphen, or "guion" in Spanish, is sometimes used to separate words in the user name or domain name.

Finally, the underscore, or "guión bajo" in Spanish, is also sometimes used to separate words in the user name or domain name.

Knowing these symbols will help you create and understand Spanish email addresses with ease. Keep them in mind next time you're communicating online in Spanish.

EXPRESSING LIKES AND DISLIKES

Next, we'll focus on expressing likes and dislikes in Spanish without delving into verb conjugation. By the end of this section, you'll be able to answer questions about your hobbies and interests and express whether you like or dislike certain things in both the singular and plural forms.

Vocabulary:

- Gustar (goos-tahr): To like
- Me gusta (meh goos-tah): I like
- Encantar (en-kahn-tahr): To love

- Odio (oh-dee-oh): I hate
- No me gusta (no meh goos-tah): I don't like

And here, you have some activities and things with which you can combine the previous phrases to explain your interests to a Spanish speaker.

- Los deportes (lohs deh-pohr-tehs): The sports
- La música (lah moo-see-kah): The music
- La comida (lah koh-mee-dah): The food
- Los animales (lohs ah-nee-mah-lehs): The animals
- La lectura (lah lehk-too-rah): The reading
- El cine (ehl see-neh): The movies/Cinema
- Los videojuegos (lohs bee-deh-oh-hweh-gohs): The video games
- Los viajes (lohs bee-ah-hehs): The travel
- La playa (lah plah-yah): The beach
- La montaña (lah mohn-tahn-yah): The mountain
- El campo (ehl kahm-poh): The countryside
- La ciudad (lah see-oo-dahd): The city

Let's see some expressions employing these words:

- Me gusta la música. (I like music.)
- Me encanta la playa. (I love the beach.)
- Odio los videojuegos. (I hate video games.)
- No me gusta la comida picante. (I don't like spicy food.)
- ¿Te gustan los deportes? (Do you like sports?)
- ¿Te encanta la lectura? (Do you love reading?)
- ¿Te gusta viajar? (Do you like to travel?)

- A mí no me gusta el cine. (I don't like movies.)

Keep in mind that if the thing being liked is plural, then you use the plural form of the verb (gustan, encantan, etc.).

By now, you have acquired a solid foundation for starting conversations in a wide range of situations in Spanish. You know how to greet and introduce yourself, ask about someone's well-being, tell time, make appointments or reservations, order food at a restaurant, understand money terminology, talk about the weather, and say hello and goodbye in different ways. Additionally, you've learned how to express your likes and dislikes, which can be extremely helpful in social settings. However, in order to become proficient Spanish speakers, we need to delve into the mechanics of the language. In the next chapter, we'll explore the fundamentals of Spanish grammar, including verb conjugation, noun and adjective agreement, and sentence structure. With these tools, you'll be able to take your Spanish conversations to a more meaningful level and communicate more effectively with native speakers. Let's go for it!

PRACTICE AND VOCABULARY

To help you practice using the phrases and vocabulary we've covered in the previous sections, I have created three different conversations between two people. However, I am going to delete one person's answers in each of these conversations, so that you can practice filling in the missing words and phrases. For each of the conversations, think about the situation and the relationship between the two speakers. Are they friends?

Colleagues? Acquaintances? This will help you choose appropriate phrases and expressions.

Conversation 1:

Person A: ¡Hola! ¿ _____?

Person B: Estoy bien, gracias. ¿Y __?

A: También estoy _____, gracias. Oye, ¿has visto la última película de acción?

B: Sí, la vi el fin de _____ pasado. Fue muy emocionante.

A: ¡Genial! ¿Te gustó?

B: Sí! Me _____ ese tipo de películas.

A: ¡A mí también! ¿Vamos a ver la nueva película de terror este fin de semana al _____?

B: Claro, me encantaría.

Conversation 2:

A: ¡_____!

B: Buen día para tí también. ¿_____?

A: Regular. Oye, ¿sabes dónde puedo encontrar un buen restaurante mexicano por aquí?

B: Sí, conozco uno que está cerca. Se _____ "El Azteca". ¿Te _____ la comida mexicana?

A: Sí. Me encanta el guacamole y los tacos.

B: Ah, entonces definitivamente deberías ir a este restaurante. Tienen los mejores tacos de la ciudad.

A: ¡Gracias por la recomendación! ¡_____!.

B: ¡Adiós!

Conversation 3:

A: ¿_____?

B: Mi nombre es Adriel. Un placer. ¿Está caluroso?

A: No. En verdad esta lloviendo mucho. ¿Te gusta este clima?

B: _____, prefiero el clima soleado.

A: ¡Yo también! _____ ir a la playa cuando hace calor.

B: Interesante, yo odio la playa, _____ ir a la montaña.

A: También amo la montaña. Pero no en verano, sino en _____, cuando esta nevado.

B: ¡Genial! Bueno, ya es tarde. Debo irme. ¡_____!

After completing the exercise, you'll have a better understanding of how to use the phrases and vocabulary we've covered in real-life conversations.

Answers:

Conversation 1:

A: Cómo estas

B: tú

A: bien

B: semana

B: encantan

A: cine

Conversation 2:

A: Buen día

B: Cómo estás

B: llama; gusta

A: Hasta luego/Adiós

Conversation 3:

A: Cómo te llamas

B: No me gusta/Lo odio

A: Me gusta

B: Yo prefiero

A: invierno

B: Adiós

GETTING COMFORTABLE WITH SPANISH GRAMMAR

Now that you have built a strong foundation with vocabulary and basic phrases, it's time to take your Spanish skills to the next level by exploring the world of grammar. Don't worry if you feel intimidated by the thought of learning grammar rules; remember the old Spanish saying, "Quien tiene boca se equivoca!", which means "Who has a mouth makes mistakes."

Making mistakes is a natural part of the learning process, and the more you practice, the better you will become. So, let's dive in and get started!

PRONOUNS

Let's start with the pronouns—the fundamental basis of every sentence.

Subject pronouns:

- Yo (yoh): I
- Tú (too): You
- Él (ehl), ella (eh-yah): He/she/it
- Nosotros/nosotras (noh-soh-trohs/noh-soh-trahs): We
- Vosotros/vosotras/ustedes (boh-soh-trohs/boh-soh-trahs/oos-teh-dehs): You (plural)
- Ellos/ellas (eh-yohs/eh-yahs): They

Possessive pronouns:

- Mío/mía (mee-oh/mee-ah): Mine
- Tuyo/tuya (too-yoh/too-yah): Yours
- Suyo/suya (soo-yoh/soo-yah): His/hers
- Nuestro/nuestra (nwes-troh/nwes-trah): Ours
- Vuestro/vuestra (bwes-troh/bwes-trah): Yours (plural)
- Suyos/suyas (soo-yohs/soo-yahs): Theirs

Direct object pronouns:

- Me (meh): Me
- Te (teh): You
- Lo/La (loh/lah): Him/it, her/it
- Nos (nohs): Us

- Os (ohs): You (plural)
- Los/Las (lohs/lahs): Them

For instance: No me gusta (I don't like it); ¡Las adoro! (I adore them); Nos vamos ahora (We are going now).

Indirect object pronouns:

- Me (meh): To me
- Te (teh): To you
- Le (leh): To him, to her, to you (formal)
- Nos (nohs): To us
- Os (ohs): To you (plural)
- Les (lehs): To them

For instance: Juan me mira (Juan looks at me); Él nos faltó el respeto (He disrespected us); ¿A vosotros no os apetece venir? (Don't you feel like coming?).

Relative pronouns:

"Los pronombres relativos" in Spanish grammar are "que," "cual," "quien," "cuyo"/"cuya," "cuanto"/"cuanta" and their plural forms.

- Que (keh): That/which/who
- Cual/cuales (khu-ahl/khu-ah-lehs): Which
- Quien/quienes (kee-ehn/kee-eh-nehs): Who/whom
- Cuyo/a, cuyos/as (khu-yoh/yah, khu-yohs/yahs): Whose/which
- Cuanto/a, cuantos/as (khu-ahn-toh/tah, khu-ahn-tohs/tahs): How much/many

Indefinite pronouns:

- Alguien (ahl-gyehn): Someone
- Nadie (nah-dyeh): No one, nobody
- Algún/alguno, algunos/as (ahl-goon/ahl-goo-noh, ahl-goo-nohs/nahs): Some (singular/plural)
- Ningún/ninguno/ninguna (neen-goon/neen-goo-noh/neen-goo-nah): None, any (singular/plural)
- Cualquier/a (kwal-kee-ehr/kwal-kee-eh-rah): Whichever
- Mucho/a, muchos/as (muh-choh/ah, muh-chohs-ahs): A lot, many
- Otro/a, otros/as (oh-troh/ah, oh-trohs/ahs): Another
- Todo/a, todos/as (toh-doh/ah, toh-dohs/ahs): All, everything
- Uno/a (uh-noh/ah): One
- Varios/as (bah-ryohs/ahs): Several, many

Demonstrative pronouns:

In English there are two words: "this" and "that." In Spanish, there are three demonstrative pronouns: Two that are the same as "this" and "that," and a third that refers to an object that is farther away.

- Este/esta (ehs-teh/ehs-tah): This
- Ese/esa (eh-seh/eh-sah): That
- Aquel/aquella (ah-kehl/ah-keh-yah): That over there

NOUNS, THEIR PLURALS, AND ARTICLES

In Spanish, there are two types of articles: definite and indefinite. The definite article corresponds to "the" in English and specifies a particular noun, while the indefinite article corresponds to "a/an" in English and refers to a nonspecific noun. Here are some examples:

- El libro (the book) - definite
- La casa (the house) - definite
- Un libro (a book) - indefinite
- Una casa (a house) - indefinite

The gender of the article must correspond to the gender of the noun it is describing. By learning the rules for noun gender and article use, you'll be able to form and understand basic Spanish sentences easily. Now, check some useful vocabulary to include in your speaking:

- El hombre (ehl ohm-breh): The man
- Un muchacho (uhn muh-chah-choh): A young man
- Las chicas (lahs chee-kahs): The girls
- Una mujer (oo-nah moo-hehr): A woman
- Los niños (lohs nee-nyohs): The children
- Una escuela (oo-nah ess-kweh-lah): A school
- Las personas (lahs pehr-soh-nahs): The people

In Spanish the plural form is determined by its last letter. The general rule for forming plurals is that we add -"s" if the noun ends in a vowel and -"es" if it ends in a consonant. Here are some examples of nouns and their plurals:

- El libro (the book) → Los libros (the books)
- La casa (the house) → Las casas (the houses)
- El árbol (the tree) → Los árboles (the trees)
- La canción (the song) → Las canciones (the songs)

To determine whether a noun is masculine or feminine, there are some general patterns to look out for. For example, most nouns that end in "o" are masculine, while most nouns that end in "a" are feminine. However, there are many exceptions to this rule, so it's best to learn the gender of a noun along with its spelling.

NOUNS AND GENDERS THAT DON'T FOLLOW THE RULES

Are you tired of learning Spanish nouns and their gender rules? Well, brace yourself because some nouns just don't follow the rules! Here are two lists of Spanish nouns with irregular gender.

Masculine nouns that end in -a:

- El día (the day)
- El agua (the water)
- El mapa (the map)
- El sofa (the sofa)
- El planeta (the planet)
- El clima (the climate)

Feminine nouns that end in -o:

- La mano (the hand)
- La radio (the radio)
- La moto (the motorcycle)
- La foto (the photo)

Now, you might be thinking, "But why do these nouns break the rules?" The truth is, there is no logical explanation. These nouns just evolved over time to have a different gender than what their endings suggest. So, the best way to learn them is through practice and repetition.

Remember, learning a language is not always logical, but it can still be fun and rewarding.

ADJECTIVES

Adjectives are a fundamental part of learning Spanish, as they are used to describe people, places, things, and ideas. Here are some of the most common adjectives you will come across:

- Feliz (feh-lees): Happy
- Triste (tree-steh): Sad
- Grande (grahn-deh): Big
- Pequeño (pek-eh-nyoh): Small
- Fuerte (foo-ehr-teh): Strong
- Débil (deh-beel): Weak
- Bonito (boh-nee-toh): Pretty
- Feo (feh-oh): Ugly

- Delgado (dehl-gah-doh): Thin
- Gordo (gohr-doh): Fat
- Inteligente (een-teh-lee-hen-teh): Intelligent
- Tonto (tohn-toh): Stupid

In Spanish, adjectives usually come after the noun they describe. However, there are some adjectives that come before the noun. Here are some rules to remember:

Adjectives of quantity or number usually come **before** the noun:

- Dos gatos negros (dohs gah-tohs neh-grohs): Two black cats
- Pocos amigos (poh-kohs ah-mee-gohs): Few friends

Adjectives of size and shape usually come **after** the noun:

- Una casa grande (oo-nah kah-sah grahn-deh): A big house
- Una mesa redonda (oo-nah meh-sah reh-dohn-dah): A round table

Adjectives of color usually come **after** the noun:

- Una camisa roja (oo-nah kah-mee-sah roh-hah): A red shirt
- Un coche azul (oon koh-cheh ah-sool): A blue car
- Un vestido blanco (oon beh-stee-doh blahn-koh): A white dress

Adjectives of personality usually come **after** the noun:

- Un hombre inteligente (oon ohm-breh een-teh-lee-hen-teh): An intelligent man
- Una pelea tonta (oo-nah peh-leh-ah tohn-tah): A stupid fight

PREPOSITIONS

Prepositions are a crucial part of any language, and Spanish has 21 prepositions in use. Let's take a look at each one and its translation, along with some examples:

- **a** (ah): to - Voy a la playa este fin de semana. (I am going to the beach this weekend.)
- **ante** (ahn-teh): before, in front of, in view of - Ante cualquier problema, llama al servicio de atención al cliente. (Before any problem, call the customer service.)
- **bajo** (bah-hoh): under, beneath, below - Los zapatos están bajo la cama. (The shoes are under the bed.)
- **con** (kohn): with - Me gusta ir al cine con mis amigos. (I like to go to the movies with my friends.)
- **contra** (kohn-trah): against - El equipo de fútbol jugó contra el equipo de baloncesto. (The soccer team played against the basketball team.)
- **de** (deh): of, from, about - La casa de mi abuela es muy grande. (My grandmother's house is very big.)
- **desde** (dehs-deh): from, since - Toco el piano desde que tenía 10 años. (I play the piano since I was 10 years old)

- **durante** (doo-rahn-teh): during - Durante el concierto, todos estaban bailando. (During the concert, everyone was dancing.)
- **en** (ehn): in, on, at - Estoy en la biblioteca estudiando para mi examen. (I am in the library studying for my exam.)
- **entre** (ehn-treh): between, among - El restaurante está entre el cine y el teatro. (The restaurant is between the movie theater and the theater.)
- **hacia** (ah-syah): towards - Caminé hacia la playa para ver el atardecer. (I walked towards the beach to see the sunset.)
- **hasta** (ahs-tah): until, up to, as far as - Caminé hasta el final de la calle. (I walked up to the end of the street.)
- **mediante** (meh-dyahn-teh): by means of, through - Se puede reservar el hotel mediante la página web. (You can book the hotel through the website.)
- **para** (pah-rah): for, in order to - Compré una tarta para el cumpleaños de mi amiga. (I bought a cake for my friend's birthday.)
- **por** (pohr): for, by, through - Hay que pronunciarse por los derechos. (You have to speak up for your rights.)
- **según** (seh-goon): according to - Según las noticias, va a llover mañana. (According to the news, it's going to rain tomorrow.)
- **sin** (seen): without - No puedo vivir sin música. (I can't live without music.)
- **sobre** (soh-breh): on, about, over - El libro trata sobre la vida de un astronauta. (The book is about the life of an astronaut.)

- **tras** (trahs): after, behind - Hay un parque tras del edificio. (There is a park behind the building.)
- **versus** (behr-soos): versus - El partido es Barcelona versus Madrid. (The game is Barcelona versus Madrid.)
- **vía** (bee-ah): via, through - El tren llega a Madrid vía Barcelona (The train arrives in Madrid via Barcelona.)

It's important to note that some verbs require specific prepositions to be used correctly. Here are some examples:

- Casarse con (kah-sahr-seh kohn): to marry [someone]
- Esperar por (eh-speh-rahr pohr): to wait for
- Hablar de (ah-blahr deh): to talk about
- Acostumbrarse a (ah-kohs-toom-brahr-seh ah): to get used to
- Depender de (deh-pehn-dehr deh): to depend on
- Soñar con (soh-nyahr kohn): to dream about
- Preguntar por (preh-goon-tahr pohr): to ask for

Learning prepositions and their corresponding verbs can be a challenge, but it's a necessary step to achieving fluency in Spanish. Remember to always study them in context and practice using them in sentences.

BASIC SENTENCE STRUCTURE

Spanish is a flexible language that allows for a lot of variation in sentence structure, but there are a few basic rules to keep in mind.

First off, let's talk about verbs. In Spanish, every verb is conjugated depending on the subject. For example, if you want to say "I cook," you would say "yo cocino." The verb "cocino" changes to match the subject pronoun "yo" (which means "I" in English). But don't worry, we'll dive deeper into verb conjugation in the next chapter.

Subject pronouns are optional in Spanish and are usually only used for emphasis. So, instead of saying "yo cocino," you could just say "cocino" to mean "I cook."

Verbs can also go before the subject for emphasis. So instead of saying "yo cocino," you would say "cocino yo" to emphasize who is doing the cooking.

Adverbs are another flexible part of Spanish sentence structure. They can go almost anywhere in a sentence, unlike in English where they usually come before the verb. For example, you could say "Rápidamente cocino la cena" (I quickly cook dinner) or "Cocino la cena rápidamente" (I cook dinner quickly).

Negative sentences require the word "no" before the verb. So, to say "I don't cook," you would say "No cocino." And don't worry, double negatives are actually the norm in Spanish, so saying "No cocino nunca" is perfectly correct, although its literal translation to English is "I don't cook never."

As I mentioned before in the book, questions in Spanish have the same structure as affirmative sentences, but with a rising intonation or by adding a tag question. For example, to ask "Do you like pizza?" you could say "¿Te gusta la pizza?" The word order is the same as in an affirmative sentence ("Te gusta la pizza"), but the rising intonation at the end makes it clear that it's a question.

As you may already notice, Spanish sentence structure is quite flexible, which allows for a lot of creativity and expression. It is a wonderful and rich language, to say the least!

In the next chapter, we'll dive into the exciting world of Spanish verbs. While it may seem daunting at first, mastering verbs is essential to becoming eloquent in Spanish. We'll start by looking at regular verbs that end in -ar, -er, and -ir. Then, we'll move on to irregular verbs and explore their unique conjugation patterns. By the end of the chapter, you'll have a solid understanding of Spanish verb conjugation and be well on your way to speaking Spanish with confidence. So, don't get discouraged, let's tackle verbs together!

PRACTICE AND VOCABULARY

1- Pronouns Quiz

A- What is the subject pronoun for "he"?

A. Yo

B. Tú

C. Él

D. Ella

B- What is the subject pronoun for "we" (all women)?

A. Nosotros
B. Nosotras
C. Ellos
D. Ellas

C- What is the possessive pronoun for "mine"?

A. Mío/mía
B. Tuyo/tuya
C. Suyo/suya
D. Nuestro/nuestra

D- What is the direct object pronoun for "her"?

A. Me
B. Te
C. Lo
D. La

Answers:

A - c)

B - b)

C - a)

D - d)

2- Fill in the blank with the correct definite article "el" or "la" (meaning "the") before the given noun. If the noun is plural, use "los" or "las" instead.

1. _____ gato (the cat)
2. _____ perro (the dog)
3. _____ casa (the house)
4. _____ coches (the cars)
5. _____ libros (the books)
6. _____ amigos (the friends)
7. _____ mesa (the table)
8. _____ silla (the chair)
9. _____ chica (the girl)
10. _____ chicos (the boys)

Answers:

1. el gato
2. el perro
3. la casa
4. los coches
5. los libros
6. los amigos
7. la mesa
8. la silla
9. la chica
10. los chicos

3- Choose an object in the room and describe it using an adjective in Spanish. Then, try to place the adjective before and after the noun to practice the placement rules.

4- Prepositions Quiz:

1. Mi hermano vive _____ California.

    a) en
    b) bajo
    c) ante
    d) con

2. Voy al gimnasio _____ mi amiga.

    a) bajo
    b) mediante
    c) hacia
    d) con

3. El libro está _____ la mesa.

    a) durante
    b) por
    c) sobre
    d) sin

4. Mi cumpleaños es _____ Diciembre.

    a) en

    b) hasta

    c) con

    d) según

5. Estamos caminando _____ el parque.

    a) hacia

    b) de

    c) contra

    d) bajo

6. El gato está escondido _____ la cama.

    a) bajo

    b) mediante

    c) con

    d) hacia

7. Shirley es alérgica _____ los mariscos.

    a) hasta

    b) a

    c) según

    d) bajo

8. Estamos yendo _____ el norte.

    a) hasta

    b) mediante

    c) hacia

    d) bajo

9. Nuestro tren está _____ la estación 4 y 6.

    a) desde

    b) durante

    c) entre

    d) contra

10. Ellos caminan _____ el césped.

    a) bajo

    b) con

    c) hacia

    d) sobre

Answers:

    1. a)

    2. d)

    3. c)

    4. a)

    5. a)

    6. a)

    7. b)

8. c)

9. c)

10. d)

5- Read and complete the sentences:

En aquel momento, eran las 2 de la _____ (1) y yo estaba disfrutando del Día de Acción de Gracias junto a mi amiga María en un restaurante del centro. En cuanto llegamos, nos sentamos en una mesa cercana a la ventana para disfrutar de la vista de la calle.

Después de unos minutos, se nos acercó un amable _____ (2). "Buenas tardes, ¿qué les gustaría pedir?" nos dijo. "¿Nos _____ (3), por favor?", le preguntamos. Él nos entregó el _____ (4) y, tras pensarlo un poco, decidimos compartir una entrada y un plato principal.

Mientras esperábamos la comida, María, intrigada, preguntó al mesero: "_____"(5). Él le respondió que contenía carne y verduras. A ella le gustaba la carne, pero _____ (6) las verduras, mientras que a mí me encanta el pescado.

Después de la deliciosa comida, María y yo hablamos sobre nuestros planes futuros. Ella me contó que le encantaría ir a la montaña, pero a mi no me gusta mucho, porque siempre está nevado y frío. "¿_____ (7) te gusta la montaña?" le pregunté. María me dijo que le gustaba la tranquilidad y los animales que se podían ver allí. Por otro lado, yo _____(8) ir a la playa y comer mariscos.

Translation:

At that time, it was 2 in the afternoon and I was enjoying Thanksgiving with my friend Maria in a downtown restaurant. As soon as we arrived, we sat at a table near the window to enjoy the view of the street.

After a few minutes, a friendly waiter approached us. "Good afternoon, what would you like to order?" He told us. "Can we get the menu, please?" we asked. He handed us the menu and, after thinking about it for a bit, we decided to share a starter and a main course.

While we were waiting for the food, María, intrigued, asked the waiter: "What's on this plate?" He replied that it contained meat and vegetables. She liked meat, but she didn't like vegetables, while I love fish.

After the delicious meal, Maria and I talked about our future plans. She told me that she would love to go to the mountains, but I don't like it very much, because it's always snowy and cold. "Why do you like the mountain?" I asked her. Maria told me that she liked the tranquility and the animals that could be seen there. On the other hand, I prefer to go to the beach and eat seafood.

Answers:

1. tarde
2. mesero
3. puede dar la carta
4. menú
5. ¿Qué lleva este plato?

6. no le gustaban
7. Por qué
8. prefiero

6- Observe and complete the following table with the gender of the nouns:

Noun	Translation	Article	Gender and Number
Allergy	Alergia	__(1)	fem. sing.
Canes	Bastones	Los	masc. pl.
Chaos	Caos	El	_____(2)
Diamonds	Diamantes	__(3)	masc. pl.
Eclipse	Eclipse	El	masc. sing.
Fissure	Fisura	La	fem. sing.
Glasses	Gafas	__(4)	fem. pl.
Hypothesis	Hipótesis	La	fem. sing.
Insects	Insectos	Los	_____(5)
Giraffes	Jirafas	Las	fem. pl.
Kermes	Kermés	__(6)	fem. sing.

Noun	Translation	Article	Gender and Number
Marble	Mármol	El	masc. sing.
Fog	Neblina	__(7)	_____(8)
Ears	Oídos	Los	masc. pl.
Pigeons	Palomas	Las	fem. pl.
Entropy	Entropía	La	fem. sing.
Butterflies	Mariposas	__(9)	fem. pl.
Keys	Llaves	Las	_____(10)
Panic	Pánico	El	masc. sing.

Answers:

1. La
2. masc. sing.
3. Los
4. Las
5. masc. pl.
6. La
7. La
8. fem. sing.
9. Las
10. fem. pl.

7- Observe the following table with masculine and feminine adjectives in the singular and in the plural:

English translation	Singular masculine	Singular feminine	Plural masculine	Plural feminine
Bitter	Amargo	Amarga	Amargos	Amargas
Careful	Cuidadoso	Cuidadosa	Cuidadosos	Cuidadosas
Clear	Claro	Clara	Claros	Claras
Dark	Oscuro	Oscura	Oscuros	Oscuras
Dirty	Sucio	Sucia	Sucios	Sucias
Easy	Fácil	Fácil	Fáciles	Fáciles
Fast	Rápido	Rápida	Rápidos	Rápidas
Fresh	Fresco	Fresca	Frescos	Frescas
Hard	Difícil	Difícil	Difíciles	Difíciles
Heavy	Pesado	Pesada	Pesados	Pesadas
High	Alto	Alta	Altos	Altas
Large	Grande	Grande	Grandes	Grandes
Light	Ligero	Ligera	Ligeros	Ligeras

English translation	Singular masculine	Singular feminine	Plural masculine	Plural feminine
Little	Pequeño	Pequeña	Pequeños	Pequeñas
Long	Largo	Larga	Largos	Largas
Low	Bajo	Baja	Bajos	Bajas
Narrow	Estrecho	Estrecha	Estrechos	Estrechas
Old	Viejo	Vieja	Viejos	Viejas
Rich	Rico	Rica	Ricos	Ricas
Short	Corto	Corta	Cortos	Cortas
Slow	Lento	Lenta	Lentos	Lentas
Small	Pequeño	Pequeña	Pequeños	Pequeñas
Strong	Fuerte	Fuerte	Fuertes	Fuertes
Tasty	Sabroso	Sabrosa	Sabrosos	Sabrosas
Thin	Delgado	Delgada	Delgados	Delgadas
Ugly	Feo	Fea	Feos	Feas
Warm	Cálido	Cálida	Cálidos	Cálidas
Wet	Mojado	Mojada	Mojados	Mojadas
White	Blanco	Blanca	Blancos	Blancas
Young	Joven	Joven	Jóvenes	Jóvenes

6

EVERY SENTENCE NEEDS A VERB

W e know that conjugating verbs in Spanish can be quite a challenge, especially for native English speakers. But fear not, as we'll start with the basics of Spanish verbs in this chapter before moving on to more complex topics like verb tenses.

As a beginner, it's important to focus on the essentials, so we won't be covering every single verb tense that exists in Spanish (there are simply too many). Instead, we'll concentrate on the verb tenses that are most useful for a beginner. These are simple and progressive tenses (past, present, and future.)

In Spanish, there are 18 tenses in total, 6 of which are simple tenses and 12 of which are compound tenses.

The six simple tenses are the present, the imperfect, the preterite, the future, the conditional, and the imperative.

Did you know that when a group of 500 Spanish learners was asked about the most challenging aspect of learning the language, 21.64% of them said that it was conjugating verbs? Only listening and understanding native speakers proved to be more difficult! (Tell Me In Spanish, n.d.). But don't let that discourage you. With practice and patience, you'll soon be able to master the intricacies of Spanish verbs.

So, let's dive into the basics of Spanish verbs and get started on our journey to verb conjugation mastery!

REGULAR VERBS IN SPANISH

Let's start at the beginning: regular verbs in the infinitive. While in English we define an infinitive by adding the preposition "to," as in "to play," in Spanish, the infinitive is identified by its three possible endings.

All regular verbs in Spanish end in -er, -ar, or -ir. It's important to remember that the verb endings will change depending on the two letters they end in and the subject pronoun. For example, let's take a look at the verbs "hablar" (to speak), "comer" (to eat), and "vivir" (to live):

Hablar:

- Yo hablo (I speak)
- Tú hablas (You speak)
- Él/Ella/Usted habla (He/She/You formal speak)
- Nosotros/Nosotras hablamos (We speak)
- Vosotros/Vosotras habláis (You all speak)
- Ellos/Ellas/Ustedes hablan (They/You all formal speak)

Comer:

- Yo como (I eat)
- Tú comes (You eat)
- Él/Ella/Usted come (He/She/You formal eat)
- Nosotros/Nosotras comemos (We eat)
- Vosotros/Vosotras coméis (You all eat)
- Ellos/Ellas/Ustedes comen (They/You all formal eat)

Vivir:

- Yo vivo (I live)
- Tú vives (You live)
- Él/Ella/Usted vive (He/She/You formal live)
- Nosotros/Nosotras vivimos (We live)
- Vosotros/Vosotras vivís (You all live)
- Ellos/Ellas/Ustedes viven (They/You all formal live)

Now, let's take a look at some common infinitive regular verbs that end in -er, -ar, or -ir:

-ar verbs:

- Hablar (ah-blahr): To speak
- Cantar (kahn-tahr): To sing
- Bailar (bahy-lahr): To dance
- Estudiar (ehs-too-dee-yahr): To study
- Escuchar (ehs-koo-chahr): To listen
- Llegar (yeh-gahr): To arrive
- Preguntar (preh-goon-tahr): To ask
- Mirar (mee-rahr): To look/watch
- Trabajar (trah-bah-hahr): To work
- Tomar (toh-mahr): To take/drink

-er verbs:

- Comer (koh-mehr): To eat
- Beber (beh-behr): To drink
- Leer (leh-ehr): To read
- Aprender (ah-preh-ndehr): To learn
- Correr (koh-rreh-r): To run
- Vender (vehn-dehr): To sell

-ir verbs:

- Vivir (bee-veer): To live
- Escribir (ehs-kree-beer): To write
- Abrir (ah-breehr): To open

- Asistir (ah-see-steer): To attend
- Partir (pahr-teer): To leave/depart

"SER" AND "ESTAR"

Are you ready to learn the difference between the Spanish verbs "ser" and "estar"? These two verbs are both translated as "to be" in English, but in Spanish, they have different meanings and uses. Let's dive in and explore the **four golden rules** of when to use each one.

The first rule is that "ser" is used for permanent characteristics, while "estar" is used for temporary states. For example, "soy aburrido" means "I am boring" as in, that is my permanent personality trait. In contrast, "estoy aburrido" means "I am bored" at the moment.

The second rule is that "ser" is used for professions and nationalities, while "estar" is used for location. For example, "soy médico" means "I am a doctor," while "estoy en casa" means "I am at home."

The third rule is that "ser" is used for descriptions and characteristics, while "estar" is used for conditions and emotions. For example, "eres inteligente" means "you are intelligent" as in, that is your permanent characteristic. On the other hand, "estás cansado" means "you are tired" at the moment.

The fourth and final rule is that "ser" is used for generalizations, while "estar" is used for specifics. For example, "la comida mexicana es picante" means "Mexican food is spicy" as a generalization, while "esta salsa está picante" means "this salsa is spicy" as a specific instance.

Now that you know the rules, let's review the conjugation of "ser" and "estar" in present simple:

Ser:

- Yo soy (yoh soh-y)
- Tú eres (too eh-rehs)
- Él/Ella/Usted es (ehl/eh-yah/oos-tehd ehs)
- Nosotros/as somos (noh-soh-trohs/as soh-mohs)
- Vosotros/as sois (voh-soh-trohs/as soh-ys)
- Ellos/Ellas/Ustedes son (eh-yohs/eh-yahs/oos-teh-dehs sohn)

Estar:

- Yo estoy (yoh eh-stoy)
- Tú estás (too eh-stahs)
- Él/Ella/Usted está (ehl/eh-yah/oos-tehd eh-stah)
- Nosotros/as estamos (noh-soh-trohs/as ehs-tah-mohs)
- Vosotros/as estáis (voh-soh-trohs/as eh-stah-ys)
- Ellos/Ellas/Ustedes están (eh-yohs/eh-yahs/oos-teh-dehs ehs-tahn)

Now you're ready to start using "ser" and "estar" like a pro! Remember to apply the four golden rules and practice a ton.

IRREGULAR VERBS

Now, let's talk about every language learner's nemesis: irregular verbs. These tricky little words don't follow the usual patterns of conjugation, and that can make them a real headache for Spanish amateurs. But fear not! Once you get the hang of them, you'll be using them like a pro.

Below, you'll find a chart with some of the most common irregular verbs and their conjugations in present simple tense. Take some time to study it, and you'll be well on your way to mastery.

Personal Pronoun	Tener (to have)	Hacer (to make)	Ir (to go)	Ver (to see)	Decir (to say)	Poder (Can)
Yo	Tengo	Hago	Voy	Veo	Digo	Puedo
Tú	Tienes	Haces	Vas	Ves	Dices	Puedes
Él/Ella/ Usted	Tiene	Hace	Va	Ve	Dice	Puede
Nosotros/ Nosotras	Tenemos	Hacemos	Vamos	Vemos	Decimos	Podemos
Vosotros/ Vosotras	Tenéis	Hacéis	Vais	Veis	Decís	Podéis
Ellos/Ellas/ Ustedes	Tienen	Hacen	Van	Ven	Dicen	Pueden

Personal Pronoun	Dar (to give)	Saber (to know facts)	Conocer (to know people)	Poner (to put)	Salir (to exit)	Traer (to bring)
Yo	Doy	Sé	Conozco	Pongo	Salgo	Traigo
Tú	Das	Sabes	Conoces	Pones	Sales	Traes
Él/Ella/ Usted	Da	Sabe	Conoce	Pone	Sale	Trae
Nosotros/ Nosotras	Damos	Sabemos	Conocemos	Ponemos	Salimos	Traemos
Vosotros/ Vosotras	Dais	Sabéis	Conocéis	Ponéis	Salís	Traéis
Ellos/Ellas/ Ustedes	Dan	Saben	Conocen	Ponen	Salen	Traen

Personal Pronoun	Venir (to come)	Oír (to hear)	Caer (to fall)	Caber (to fit)	Jugar (to play)	Cerrar (to close)
Yo	Vengo	Oigo	Caigo	Quepo	Juego	Cierro
Tú	Vienes	Oyes	Caes	Cabes	Juegas	Cierras
Él/Ella/ Usted	Viene	Oye	Cae	Cabe	Juega	Cierra
Nosotros/ Nosotras	Venimos	Oímos	Caemos	Cabemos	Jugamos	Cerramos
Vosotros/ Vosotras	Venís	Oís	Caéis	Cabéis	Jugáis	Cerráis
Ellos/Ellas/ Ustedes	Vienen	Oyen	Caen	Caben	Juegan	Cierran

Personal Pronoun	Empezar (to begin)	Entender (to understand)	Pensar (to think)	Perder (to lose)	Sentir (to feel)
Yo	Empiezo	Entiendo	Pienso	Pierdo	Siento
Tú	Empiezas	Entiendes	Piensas	Pierdes	Sientes
Él/Ella/ Usted	Empieza	Entiende	Piensa	Pierde	Siente
Nosotros/ Nosotras	Empezamos	Entendemos	Pensamos	Perdemos	Sentimos
Vosotros/ Vosotras	Empezáis	Entendéis	Pensáis	Perdéis	Sentís
Ellos/Ellas/ Ustedes	Empiezan	Entienden	Piensan	Pierden	Sienten

Personal Pronoun	Costar (to cost)	Lastimar (to hurt)	Encontrar (to find)	Oler (to smell)
Yo	Cuesto	Lastimo	Encuentro	Huelo
Tú	Cuestas	Lastimas	Encuentras	Hueles
Él/Ella/ Usted	Cuesta	Lastima	Encuentra	Huele
Nosotros/ Nosotras	Costamos	Lastimamos	Encontramos	Olemos
Vosotros/ Vosotras	Costáis	Lastimáis	Encontráis	Oléis
Ellos/Ellas/ Ustedes	Cuestan	Lastiman	Encuentran	Huelen

Personal Pronoun	Recordar (to remember)	Conseguir (to get)	Elegir (to choose)	Pedir (to ask for)
Yo	Recuerdo	Consigo	Elijo	Pido
Tú	Recuerdas	Consigues	Eliges	Pides
Él/Ella/ Usted	Recuerda	Consigue	Elige	Pide
Nosotros/ Nosotras	Recordamos	Conseguimos	Elegimos	Pedimos
Vosotros/ Vosotras	Recordáis	Conseguís	Elegís	Pedís
Ellos/Ellas/ Ustedes	Recuerdan	Consiguen	Eligen	Piden

THE SIMPLE TENSES

Now, it is time to talk about the simple tenses in Spanish. Don't worry, it's as simple as it sounds. We'll start by discussing regular verbs. They are, naturally, much easier to conjugate than irregular verbs because they follow the same patterns.

Regarding the present simple, we have used it to exemplify the conjugation of verbs throughout the book: For example, when we talk about regular and irregular verbs, we conjugate the verb "hablar" (to speak) in the present simple: "yo hablo," "tu hablas," "el/ella habla..."

Here are the conjugations for the regular verb **"hablar"** in the simple past and simple future:

Simple Past:

- Yo hablé (ah-bleh): I spoke
- Tú hablaste (ah-blas-teh): You spoke
- Él/ella/usted habló (ah-bloh): He/she/you (formal) spoke
- Nosotros/nosotras hablamos (ah-blah-mohs): We spoke
- Vosotros/vosotras hablasteis (ah-blas-tays): You all spoke
- Ellos/ellas/ustedes hablaron (ah-blah-ron): They/you all (formal) spoke

Simple Future:

- Yo hablaré (ah-blah-reh): I will speak
- Tú hablarás (ah-blah-rahs): You will speak
- Él/ella/usted hablará (ah-blah-rah): He/she/you (formal) will speak
- Nosotros/nosotras hablaremos (ah-blah-reh-mohs): We will speak
- Vosotros/vosotras hablaréis (ah-blah-reh-ees): You all will speak
- Ellos/ellas/ustedes hablarán (ah-blah-rahn): They/you all (formal) will speak

Here, I present a chart with the **past simple** conjugations of the most common regular verbs:

Personal Pronoun	Hablar (to talk)	Comer (to eat)	Vivir (to live)	Bailar (to dance)	Estudiar (to study)
Yo	hablé	comí	viví	bailé	estudié
Tú	hablaste	comiste	viviste	bailaste	estudiaste
Él/Ella/ Usted	habló	comió	vivió	bailó	estudió
Nosotros/ Nosotras	hablamos	comimos	vivimos	bailamos	estudiamos
Vosotros/ Vosotras	hablasteis	comisteis	vivisteis	bailasteis	estudiasteis
Ellos/Ellas/ Ustedes	hablaron	comieron	vivieron	bailaron	estudiaron

Personal Pronoun	Trabajar (to work)	Tomar (to take/to drink)	Cantar (to sing)	Caminar (to walk)	Viajar (to travel)
Yo	trabajé	tomé	canté	caminé	viajé
Tú	trabajaste	tomaste	cantaste	caminaste	viajaste
Él/Ella/ Usted	trabajó	tomó	cantó	caminó	viajó
Nosotros/ Nosotras	trabajamos	tomamos	cantamos	caminamos	viajamos
Vosotros/ Vosotras	trabajasteis	tomasteis	cantasteis	caminasteis	viajasteis
Ellos/Ellas/ Ustedes	trabajaron	tomaron	cantaron	caminaron	viajaron

Now, observe how the same verbs are conjugated in the **simple future**:

Personal Pronoun	Hablar (to talk)	Comer (to eat)	Vivir (to live)	Bailar (to dance)	Estudiar (to study)
Yo	hablaré	comeré	viviré	bailaré	estudiaré
Tú	hablarás	comerás	vivirás	bailarás	estudiarás
Él/Ella/ Usted	hablará	comerá	vivirá	bailará	estudiará
Nosotros/ Nosotras	hablaremos	comeremos	viviremos	bailaremos	estudiaremos
Vosotros/ Vosotras	hablaréis	comeréis	viviréis	bailaréis	estudiaréis
Ellos/Ellas/ Ustedes	hablarán	comerán	vivirán	bailarán	estudiarán

Personal Pronoun	Trabajar (to work)	Tomar (to take/to drink)	Cantar (to sing)	Caminar (to walk)	Viajar (to travel)
Yo	trabajaré	tomaré	cantaré	caminaré	viajaré
Tú	trabajarás	tomarás	cantarás	caminarás	viajarás
Él/Ella/ Usted	trabajará	tomará	cantará	caminará	viajará
Nosotros/ Nosotras	trabajaremos	tomaremos	cantaremos	caminaremos	viajaremos
Vosotros/ Vosotras	trabajaréis	tomaréis	cantaréis	caminaréis	viajaréis
Ellos/Ellas/ Ustedes	trabajarán	tomarán	cantarán	caminarán	viajarán

Lastly, we have irregular verbs. These verbs don't follow regular patterns, so you'll need to memorize their conjugations. Here are some of the most common irregular verbs in **simple past**:

Personal Pronoun	Ser (to be)	Estar (to be)	Tener (to have)	Querer (to want)
Yo	Fui	Estuve	Tuve	Quise
Tú	Fuiste	Estuviste	Tuviste	Quisiste
Él/Ella/Usted	Fue	Estuvo	Tuvo	Quiso
Nosotros/Nosotras	Fuimos	Estuvimos	Tuvimos	Quisimos
Vosotros/Vosotras	Fuisteis	Estuvisteis	Tuvisteis	Quisisteis
Ellos/Ellas/Ustedes	Fueron	Estuvieron	Tuvieron	Quisieron

Personal Pronoun	Hacer (to do)	Ir (to go)	Venir (to come)	Decir (to say)
Yo	Hice	Fui	Vine	Dije
Tú	Hiciste	Fuiste	Viniste	Dijiste
Él/Ella/Usted	Hizo	Fue	Vino	Dijo
Nosotros/Nosotras	Hicimos	Fuimos	Vinimos	Dijimos
Vosotros/Vosotras	Hicisteis	Fuisteis	Vinisteis	Dijisteis
Ellos/Ellas/Ustedes	Hicieron	Fueron	Vinieron	Dijeron

Here, you have a chart with the same irregular verbs conjugated in **simple future**:

Personal Pronoun	Ser (to be)	Estar (to be)	Tener (to have)	Querer (to want)
Yo	Seré	Estaré	Tendré	Querré
Tú	Serás	Estarás	Tendrás	Querrás
Él/Ella/Usted	Será	Estará	Tendrá	Querrá
Nosotros/Nosotras	Seremos	Estaremos	Tendremos	Querremos
Vosotros/Vosotras	Seréis	Estaréis	Tendréis	Querréis
Ellos/Ellas/ Ustedes	Serán	Estarán	Tendrán	Querrán

Personal Pronoun	Hacer (to do)	Ir (to go)	Venir (to come)	Decir (to say)
Yo	Haré	Iré	Vendré	Diré
Tú	Harás	Irás	Vendrás	Dirás
Él/Ella/Usted	Hará	Irá	Vendrá	Dirá
Nosotros/Nosotras	Haremos	Iremos	Vendremos	Diremos
Vosotros/Vosotras	Haréis	Iréis	Vendréis	Diréis
Ellos/Ellas/ Ustedes	Harán	Irán	Vendrán	Dirán

The two most important verbs in Spanish: "ser" and "estar." They both mean "to be" and now we will learn when we are supposed to use each of them. I mentioned these verbs before and now we'll look at them in more detail.

These are both irregular verbs, which means they don't follow regular conjugation patterns. "Ser" is used to talk about permanent or long-term characteristics, while "estar" is used to talk about temporary states or conditions.

Here are the conjugations of the verb "**ser**" in the simple past and simple future:

Simple past:

- Yo fui (fwee): I was
- Tú fuiste (fwis-teh): You were
- Él/ella/usted fue (fweh): He/she/you (formal) was
- Nosotros/nosotras fuimos (fwee-mohs): We were
- Vosotros/vosotras fuisteis (fwee-stays): You all were
- Ellos/ellas/ustedes fueron (fweh-ron): They/you all (formal) were

Simple future:

- Yo seré (seh-reh): I will be
- Tú serás (seh-rahs): You will be
- Él/ella/usted será (seh-rah): He/she/you (formal) will be
- Nosotros/nosotras seremos (seh-reh-mohs): We will be
- Vosotros/vosotras seréis (seh-reh-ees): You all will be

- Ellos/ellas/ustedes serán (seh-rahn): They/you all (formal) will be

If you have any doubts about the pronunciation of the letter "r" in these words, take a quick look at the first chapter, where we addressed its correct pronunciation.

Here are the conjugations of the Spanish verb "**estar**" in the simple past and simple future tenses:

Simple past:

- Yo estuve (ehs-too-veh)
- Tú estuviste (ehs-too-vees-teh)
- Él/Ella/Usted estuvo (ehs-too-boh)
- Nosotros/Nosotras estuvimos (ehs-too-vee-mohs)
- Vosotros/Vosotras estuvisteis (ehs-too-vees-tays)
- Ellos/Ellas/Ustedes estuvieron (ehs-too-byeh-rohn)

Simple future:

- Yo estaré (ehs-tah-reh)
- Tú estarás (ehs-tah-rahs)
- Él/Ella/Usted estará (ehs-tah-rah)
- Nosotros/Nosotras estaremos (ehs-tah-reh-mohs)
- Vosotros/Vosotras estaréis (ehs-tah-reys)
- Ellos/Ellas/Ustedes estarán (ehs-tah-rahn)

Remember: "Yo fui" means "I was" and "yo estuve" also means "I was" in Spanish, but the first one is used for permanent states and "yo estuve" is used for temporary states. Similarly, "yo seré" and "yo estaré" both mean "I will be" in Spanish. In the same way, the first one is used for permanent situations while the second one is used for temporary situations. If you need a reminder of how to correctly use these two important verbs, just go back quickly to check the golden rules!

Here you have some examples:

- Yo estuve de vacaciones en los Estados Unidos cuando tenía 7 años. (I was on vacation in the United States when I was 7 years old.)
- Yo fui el presidente de mi clase dos años consecutivos. (I was the president of my class two years in a row).
- Tú serás el mejor de tu clase. (You will be the best in your class).
- Mis padres estarán de viaje el próximo mes. (My parents will be traveling next month).

THE PROGRESSIVE TENSES

Are you ready to take your Spanish skills to the next level? Then let's talk about the progressive tenses.

First, let's clarify the difference between the present participle and the gerund. In English, the present participle is used with the verb "to be" to describe actions that are happening in the moment or near future, for example, "I am learning," or "I am going there next weekend."

The gerund, on the other hand, is a noun and can be used as the subject or object of a sentence, for example, "Swimming is fun" or

"She loves swimming."

In Spanish, both the present participle and the gerund are referred to as "gerundio." The present participle or gerund in Spanish is formed by adding "-ando" or "-iendo" to the stem of the verb, for example, "hablando" (talking) or "comiendo" (eating). It can be used in the same way as in English, to describe actions that are happening at the moment, for example, "Estoy hablando" (I am talking).

As in English, it can function as an object. For example, "Caminando se llega lejos" (Walking gets you far). In this example, the nuclear verb is "llega" (arrive). That's the action the subject does. "Caminando" is the object, in the sense that it is a means to arrive "lejos" (far).

So, the gerund in Spanish is rather an action taking place in the present moment ("Estoy hablando") or an object (Hablando se entiende la gente.)

And here are some examples of verbs in their gerund form:

- Com**iendo** (koh-mee-ehn-doh): Eating
- Camin**ando** (kah-mee-nahn-doh): Walking
- Escrib**iendo** (eh-skree-bee-ehn-doh): Writing

But what if the verb (from -"er" and -"ir" group) has a **vowel before the termination**? In this case, you just add -"yendo." For example, the present participle of "leer" (to read) is "leyendo" (reading), and the present participle of "const**ruir**" (to build) is "construyendo" (building).

- Ir (eer): Yendo (going) - Exception
- **Oír** (oh-eer): Oyendo (hearing) - Add "yendo" since there's a vowel before the termination "ir."
- Decir (deh-seer): Diciendo (saying) - Add "iendo" since there's a consonant before the termination "ir."
- Hacer (ah-sehr): Haciendo (doing) - Add "iendo" since there's a consonant before the termination "er."
- **Ser** (sehr): Siendo (being) - Add "iendo" since there's a consonant before the termination "er."
- Ve**n**ir (beh-neer): Viniendo (coming) - Add "iendo" since there's a consonant before the termination "ir."

However, not all verbs follow this pattern. Some of them have irregular present participles. You'll learn them by practicing and the more you get familiar with the language, the more you'll be able to identify exceptions.

Now that you know how to form present participles, you can use them to create the present progressive tense, also known as the present continuous tense. This tense is used to describe an action that is currently in progress.

To form the present progressive tense in Spanish, you need to use the verb "estar" (to be) in the present tense, followed by the present participle of the verb you want to use. For example, "I am eating" would be "Estoy comiendo" (ess-toy coh-mee-en-doh).

You can also use the past and future progressive tenses by using the imperfect and future tenses of "estar," respectively, followed by the present participle of the verb. For example, "I was eating" would be "Estaba comiendo" (ess-tah-bah coh-mee-en-doh), and

"I will be eating" would be "Estaré comiendo" (ess-tah-reh coh-mee-en-doh).

Let me give you some examples:

- Estoy hablando por teléfono. (I am talking on the phone.)
- Estábamos caminando por el parque cuando empezó a llover. (We were walking in the park when it started raining.)
- Voy a estar estudiando para mi examen toda la noche. (I am going to be studying for my exam all night.)
- Está bailando muy bien. (He/She is dancing very well.)
- Estuvieron durmiendo toda la tarde después de la fiesta. (They were sleeping all afternoon after the party.)

You may be thinking that the present progressive is the same and indistinguishable from the gerund or participle. Let me briefly explain the difference:

In both Spanish and English, the gerund or participle is the word that ends in "ando/iendo" for Spanish, or "ing" in English. Meanwhile, the present progressive is the grammatical construction that indicates an event that is taking place in the present.

The sentence "estamos comiendo" (we are eating) is in the present progressive, where the gerund/participle is "comiendo." But the sentence could be also conjugated in the past progressive: "estabamos comiendo" (we were eating), and the gerund/participle would remain the same: "comiendo."

So, practice forming present participles and using them in the present, past, and future progressive tenses to take your Spanish verb conjugation skills to the next level!

TENER: VERB AND PHRASES

Next, we are going to talk about one of the most important and versatile verbs in the Spanish language, "tener." This verb has many uses beyond just meaning "to have," which is its most common translation. Let's explore some of the different ways to use it.

Firstly, let's look at some common expressions with "tener":

- Tener hambre (teh-ner ahm-breh): to be hungry
- Tener sed (teh-ner sehd): to be thirsty
- Tener frío/calor (teh-ner free-oh/kah-lohr): to be cold/hot
- Tener miedo (teh-ner mee-eh-doh): to be afraid
- Tener sueño (teh-ner sweh-nyoh): to be sleepy

Another important use of this verb is to express age:

- Tengo veinticinco años (tehn-goh veh-een-tee-seen-coh ahn-yohs): I am twenty-five years old.

Finally, let's talk about "tener que" (teh-ner keh), which means "to have to" or "must" in English. This phrase is used to express obligation or necessity.

For example:

- Tengo que estudiar (tehn-goh keh eh-stoo-dee-ahr): I have to study.
- No tengo que trabajar mañana (noh tehn-goh keh trah-bah-jahr mah-nyah-nah): I don't have to work tomorrow.
- ¿Tienes que ir al médico? (tyeh-nes keh eer ahl meh-dee-koh): Do you have to go to the doctor?

Remember, this is a very important verb in Spanish, not only to express possession, but also to talk about feelings, age, and obligations.

By now, you've probably noticed that Spanish verbs can be a bit of a challenge to master, but don't worry, I'm here to help you understand the perfect tenses.

To form the perfect tenses, you'll need to use the auxiliary verb "haber" and the past participle of the main verb. But wait, what is "haber"? You might remember that haber is one of the translations for "have" in Spanish, but when used as an auxiliary verb, it means "have" in the sense of "have done something."

THE PERFECT TENSES

Let's take a look at how to conjugate haber in the indicative present, imperfect, and future tenses:

- **Indicative present:** he, has, ha, hemos, habéis, han
- **Indicative imperfect:** había, habías, había, habíamos, habíais, habían

- **Indicative future**: habré, habrás, habrá, habremos, habréis, habrán

Now, let's move on to the past participle. In Spanish, there are two different sets of past participles, depending on the last two letters of the verb.

1. Verbs that end in -"**ar**": The past participle is formed by replacing -"ar" with -"**ado**":

- "hablar" (ah-blahr) becomes "hablado" (ah-blah-doh) (spoken)
- "caminar" (kah-mee-nahr) becomes "caminado" (kah-mee-nah-doh) (walked)
- "cantar" (kahn-tahr) becomes "cantado" (kahn-tah-doh) (sung)
- "estudiar" (ehs-too-dee-ahr) becomes "estudiado" (ehs-too-dee-ah-doh) (studied)
- "mirar" (mee-rahr) becomes "mirado" (mee-rah-doh) (watched)
- "nadar" (nah-dahr) becomes "nadado" (nah-dah-doh) (swam)
- "jugar" (hoo-gahr) becomes "jugado" (hoo-gah-doh) (played)
- "bailar" (bahy-lahr) becomes "bailado" (bahy-lah-doh) (danced)
- "viajar" (byah-hahr) becomes "viajado" (byah-hah-doh) (traveled)
- "cocinar" (koh-see-nahr) becomes "cocinado" (koh-see-nah-doh) (cooked)

2. Verbs that end in -"er" or -"ir": The past participle is formed by replacing them with -"**ido**."

- "comer" (koh-mehr) becomes "comido" (koh-mee-doh) (eaten)
- "vivir" (bee-beer) becomes "vivido" (bee-bee-doh) (lived)
- "beber" (beh-behr) becomes "bebido" (beh-bee-doh) (drunk)
- "correr" (koh-rreh-r) becomes "corrido" (koh-ree-doh) (run)
- "leer" (leh-ehr) becomes "leído" (leh-ee-doh) (read)
- "decidir" (deh-see-deer) becomes "decidido" (deh-see-dee-doh) (decided)
- "partir" (pahr-teer) becomes "partido" (pahr-tee-doh) (divided)
- "recibir" (reh-see-beer) becomes "recibido" (reh-see-bee-doh) (received)
- "subir" (soo-beer) becomes "subido" (soo-bee-doh) (gone up)
- "salir" (sah-leer) becomes "salido" (sah-lee-doh) (gone out)

Now that you know how to form the past participle, it's time to learn about some common irregular past participles in Spanish.

Here are some of the most common ones:

- "cubrir" (koo-breer) becomes "cubierto" (koo-bee-ehr-toh) (covered)
- "decir" (deh-seer) becomes "dicho" (dee-choh) (said)

- "escribir" (eh-skree-beer) becomes "escrito" (eh-skree-toh) (written)
- "hacer" (ah-sehr) becomes "hecho" (eh-choh) (done/made)
- "morir" (moh-reer) becomes "muerto" (moo-ehr-toh) (died)
- "poner" (poh-neer) becomes "puesto" (poo-ehs-toh) (put)
- "romper" (rohm-pehr) becomes "roto" (roh-toh) (broken)
- "ver" (vehr) becomes "visto" (vee-stoh) (seen)
- "volver" (vohl-vehr) becomes "vuelto" (voo-ehl-toh) (returned)

Now that you have a better understanding of the perfect tenses in Spanish, it's time to start practicing! Try forming some sentences using the perfect tenses with different verbs and subjects based on the following examples:

- Juan ha corrido una maratón. (Juan has run a marathon.)
- Mis hermanas habían decidido ir a la fiesta. (My sisters had decided to go to the party.)
- En los próximos meses, habrás escrito un libro. (In the next few months, you will have written a book.)

Good luck!

REFLEXIVE VERBS

Let's move on to the last topic (I promise) related to conjugations and tenses in Spanish: reflexive verbs.

Reflexive verbs are verbs that are used to indicate that the action is being performed on oneself. In other words, the subject is performing the action to or for themselves. This is done by adding a reflexive pronoun before the verb. There are six reflexive pronouns in Spanish:

- me
- te
- se
- nos
- os
- se

The reflexive pronoun used will depend on the subject performing the action. For example, if the subject is "yo" (I), the reflexive pronoun used would be "me." If the subject is "él" (he), the reflexive pronoun used would be "se."

Reflexive pronouns can be placed before the verb or can be attached to the end of an infinitive verb or present participle. For example, "me lavo" (I wash myself) or "lavarme" (to wash myself).

Reflexive verbs can be grouped into three categories:

Daily routine actions such as bathing, getting dressed, and brushing teeth.

- Levantarse (leh-bahn-TAHR-seh): To get up
- Ducharse (doo-CHAHR-seh): To take a shower
- Maquillarse (mah-kee-YAHHR-seh): To put on makeup

Actions performed on **parts of the body**.

- Peinarse (peh-ee-NAHR-seh): To comb one's hair
- Afeitarse (ah-fay-TAHR-seh): To shave
- Pintarse las uñas (peen-TAHR-seh lahs OO-nyahs): To paint one's nails

Actions done **for oneself** or **to oneself**.

- Acordarse (ah-kor-DAHR-seh): To remember
- Sentarse (sehn-TAHR-seh): To sit down
- Divertirse (dee-vehr-TEER-seh): To have fun

I know: you feel lost. You think that Spanish is too overwhelming and that you will never be able to learn all those tenses and conjugations. I understand you because, believe it or not, even for Spanish speakers it is complicated! How many times has my Spanish teacher corrected me in class for misconjugating the verbs in my sentences? In my own mother tongue!

But don't be discouraged. Learning a language is a task that requires a lot of commitment and energy, not for nothing it takes us at least the first six years of our lives to learn to communicate effectively in our mother tongue.

Let me tell you a story about someone like you, who felt the same way you are feeling now about learning Spanish. His name is Carl.

Carl is a language learner who was feeling completely overwhelmed by the vast number of Spanish verbs to learn. He couldn't believe that even the most basic verbs like "am," "are," and "is" had 12 different forms in the present tense alone! Carl was feeling defeated and frustrated, thinking that he would never be able to master the language.

But he was determined not to give up. He decided to take matters into his own hands and come up with a creative solution. He created color-coded flashcards for each verb tense and recorded himself saying different conjugations of the verbs. This way, he could listen to the recordings while he went about his daily routine, doing chores or commuting to work.

Slowly but surely, Carl started to see improvement. He could recognize patterns in verb conjugations and was able to use the correct form more often. He no longer felt overwhelmed, and he was excited to see how much more he could improve.

Carl's experience is relatable to many language learners who feel overwhelmed by the complexity of Spanish verbs. But with determination, creativity, and a little bit of hard work, anyone can master these tricky language elements.

Throughout this chapter, you have explored all the important verb conjugations to be able to express yourself profoundly in Spanish.

On this path, social faux pas can be detrimental to our confidence, but with an appreciation for Spanish culture, we can better understand and communicate with Spanish people. By finding common ground and conversation starters, we can create meaningful connections and improve our language skills. In the final chapter, we will delve deeper into Spanish culture and customs, and how they impact the language. Stay tuned for more insights and tips on mastering Spanish!

PRACTICE AND VOCABULARY

1- Order the following sentences:

1. los/ juega / mi hermano / videojuegos

---

2. voy / tarde / a / la universidad / siempre

---

3. los pájaros /cantan / en / árboles / los

---

4. habla / ella / con / su amiga / por teléfono

---

5. un libro / leemos / en la biblioteca / nosotros

---

6. nosotros / prepara / mi madre / la cena / para

_____

7. corren / niños / en el parque / los

_____

8. escucha / él/ en su habitación / la música

_____

9. trabajan / maestros / en la escuela / los

_____

10. el perro / en el jardín / su comida / siempre / come

_____

Answers:

1. Mi hermano juega los videojuegos. (My brother plays video games.)
2. Siempre voy tarde a la universidad. (I'm always late for university.)
3. Los pájaros cantan en los árboles. (The birds sing in the trees.)
4. Ella habla con su amiga por teléfono. (She talks to her friend on the phone.)
5. Nosotros leemos un libro en la biblioteca. (We read a book in the library.)
6. Mi madre prepara la cena para nosotros. (My mother prepares dinner for us.)

7. Los niños corren en el parque. (The children run in the park.)
8. Él escucha la música en su habitación. (He listens to music in his room.)
9. Los maestros trabajan en la escuela. (The teachers work at the school.)
10. El perro come su comida siempre en el jardín. (The dog always eats his food in the garden.)

2- Conjugate the following verbs in the simple tenses with the correct pronoun, either "ser" or "estar":

1. Yo _____ en casa. (estar; past)
2. Ella _____ muy simpática. (ser; present)
3. Tú _____ de España, ¿verdad? (ser; present)
4. Nosotros _____ en la playa. (estar; future)
5. Vosotros _____ muy cansados. (estar; past)
6. Ustedes _____ mis amigos. (ser; present)
7. Él no _____ muy feliz. (estar; past)
8. Yo no _____ seguro. (estar; future)
9. Ellas _____ enfermas. (estar; future)
10. Usted _____ muy amable conmigo. (ser; present)

Answers:

1. estuve
2. es
3. eres
4. estaremos
5. estuvisteis

6. son
7. estuvo
8. estaré
9. estarán
10. es

3- Complete the following sentences with the correct form of the verb in parentheses in the progressive tense:

1. Yo _____ (hablar) con mi amigo en este momento. (present)
2. Tú _____ (bailar) en la fiesta de anoche. (past)
3. Él _____ (comer) en el restaurante a las ocho de la noche. (past)
4. Nosotros _____ (estudiar) en la biblioteca hoy en la tarde. (present)
5. Vosotros _____ (leer) el libro en este momento. (present)
6. Ellos _____ (jugar) al fútbol todos los sábados. (present)
7. Yo _____ (cantar) en el karaoke con mis amigos mañana por la noche. (future)
8. Tú y yo _____ (bailar) en la discoteca la próxima semana. (future)
9. Ella _____ (ver) la televisión a esta hora. (present)
10. Ustedes _____ (escribir) un correo electrónico en este momento. (present)

Answers:

1. estoy hablando
2. estuviste bailando
3. estuvo comiendo
4. estamos estudiando
5. estáis leyendo
6. están jugando
7. estaré cantando
8. estaremos bailando
9. está viendo
10. están escribiendo

4- Translate the following sentences into Spanish. I added the verbal tense and number to make it easier for you to identify the correct translation:

1. I have a dog. (Present simple)

_____

2. They will have a party next week. (Future simple)

_____

3. She had a headache yesterday. (Past simple)

_____

4. You have a lot of books. (Present simple, plural)

_____

5. We will have to work late tonight. (Future simple, plural)

_____

6. He had a nice car when he was young. (Past simple)

_____

7. I have to study for the exam. (Present simple)

_____

8. She will have a baby in a few months. (Future simple)

_____

9. They have a great relationship. (Present simple, plural)

_____

10. I had a good time at the party last night. (Past simple)

_____

Answers:

1. Tengo un perro.
2. Tendrán una fiesta la próxima semana.
3. Ella tuvo dolor de cabeza ayer.
4. Tienes muchos libros.
5. Tendremos que trabajar hasta tarde esta noche.
6. Él tuvo un coche bonito cuando era joven.
7. Tengo que estudiar para el examen.
8. Ella tendrá un bebé en unos meses.
9. Ellos tienen una gran relación.
10. Me divertí en la fiesta anoche.

5- Read and complete the translation:

Estaba navegando en mi barco hacia una isla desconocida, cuando de repente una tormenta se desató y el mar comenzó a agitarse violentamente. Mientras luchaba por mantener el rumbo, mi brújula se rompió y perdí toda noción de la dirección. Después de varias horas de luchar contra los elementos, finalmente avisté una costa rocosa y decidí atracar mi barco en la playa.

Una vez en tierra, empecé a explorar la isla y me di cuenta de que estaba completamente desierta. No había señales de vida humana en ninguna parte, pero encontré una cueva oculta en una colina cercana. Decidí investigar y encontré una cámara secreta llena de tesoros antiguos, pero también descubrí que la isla estaba habitada por una tribu de nativos hostiles.

A medida que exploraba más, encontré un mapa que mostraba la ubicación de un tesoro aún mayor. Sin embargo, pronto me di cuenta de que estaba siendo perseguido por los nativos. Luché por mi vida para escapar de aquella selvática jungla y regresar a mi barco, pero nunca olvidaré mi aventura en esa misteriosa isla solitaria.

Ahora, de vuelta en mi hogar, me pregunto qué habría pasado si hubiera permanecido más tiempo en la isla. ¿Habría encontrado el tesoro y escapado de los nativos? ¿O habría sido capturado y convertido en su prisionero para siempre? Todavía me pregunto qué secretos más podría haber descubierto en esa isla misteriosa.

Mirando hacia el futuro, me doy cuenta de que nunca sabré la respuesta a esas preguntas. Pero eso no significa que deba dejar de explorar y descubrir nuevos lugares. La próxima vez que zarpe hacia lo desconocido, estaré mejor preparado para enfrentar cualquier desafío que se presente. Quién sabe qué aventuras esperan en el horizonte, pero estoy listo para descubrirlas.

Translation:

I was sailing on my ship to an _____ _____ (1), when suddenly a storm _____(2) and the sea _____ ___ ___(3) violently. As I struggled to _____(4) on course, my compass broke and __ _____(5) all sense of direction. After several hours of fighting the elements, I finally spotted a rocky shoreline and decided to dock my boat on the _____(6).

Once on land, I began __ _____ (7) the island and realized that it was completely deserted. There were no signs of human life anywhere, but I __ _____ (8) a hidden cave in a nearby hill. I decided to investigate and found a secret chamber full of ancient treasures, but also _____(9) that the island was inhabited by a tribe of hostile natives.

As I explored further, __ _____ _____ (10) a map that showed the location of an even bigger treasure. However, I _____ (11) realized that I was being persecuted by the natives. I fought for my life to escape from that jungle and return to my ship, but I _____ (12) never forget my adventure on that mysterious lonely island.

Now, back home, I wonder what _____ _____ (13) happened if I had stayed longer on the island. Would I have found the treasure and escaped from the natives? Or would I have been _____ (14) and made their prisoner forever? I still wonder what more secrets I could have _____ (15) on that mysterious island.

_____ (16) to the future, I realize that I will never _____ __ _____(17) to those questions. But that doesn't mean I should stop exploring and discovering new places. The next time I set sail into the unknown, ____ _____(18) be better prepared to face any challenge that comes my way. Who knows what adventures await on the horizon, but I'm ready to discover them.

Answers:

1. unknown island
2. broke out
3. began to rage
4. stay
5. I lost
6. beach
7. to explore
8. did find
9. Discovered
10. I came across
11. soon
12. will
13. would have
14. captured
15. discovered
16. Looking

17. know the answer
18. I will

6- To expand and complete your vocabulary, you will need adverbs. Observe the following table with adverbs of place, time, manner, quantity, affirmation, negation, and doubt:

Category (Categoría)	Adverb (Adverbio)
Place (Lugar)	aquí (here), allí (there), ahí (there), arriba (up), abajo (down), adentro (inside), afuera (outside), lejos (far), cerca (near)
Time (Tiempo)	ahora (now), antes (before), después (after), temprano (early), tarde (late), pronto (soon), ya (already), todavía (still), nunca (never)
Manner (Modo)	bien (well), mal (badly), lentamente (slowly), rápidamente (quickly), suavemente (softly), fuertemente (strongly), fácilmente (easily), difícilmente (difficultly), claramente (clearly)

Category (Categoría)	Adverb (Adverbio)
Quantity (Cantidad)	mucho (much/many), poco (little/few), más (more), menos (less), demasiado (too much), suficiente (enough), casi (almost), apenas (hardly), todo (all/everything)
Affirmation (Afirmación)	sí (yes), ciertamente (certainly), claro (of course), efectivamente (indeed), verdaderamente (truly), obviamente (obviously), también (also), incluso (even), siempre (always)
Negation (Negación)	no (no), nunca (never), jamás (never), tampoco (neither), ningún (none), nada (nothing), nadie (nobody), apenas (barely/hardly)
Doubt (Duda)	quizás (perhaps), tal vez (maybe), posiblemente (possibly), acaso (possibly), quizá (maybe), seguramente (surely), probablemente (probably), realmente (really), casi (almost)

Usage examples:

- Voy a dejar el libro **aquí**. (I'm going to leave the book here.)
- Mañana **temprano** tengo una reunión importante. (Early tomorrow I have an important meeting.)
- La música sonaba **suavemente** en el fondo. (The music was playing softly in the background.)
- Comí **demasiado** y ahora me siento mal. (I ate too much and now I feel sick.)
- Sí, **definitivamente** quiero ir contigo. (Yes, I definitely want to go with you.)

- No, **nunca** he estado en ese restaurante. (No, I've never been to that restaurant.)
- **Tal vez** deberíamos llamar a alguien para que nos ayude. (Maybe we should call someone to help us.)
- **Quizás** ella tenga la respuesta que estamos buscando. (Perhaps she has the answer we're looking for.)
- **Probablemente** lleguemos **tarde** si no nos apuramos. (We'll probably be late if we don't hurry.)
- **Realmente no** entiendo lo que está pasando. (I really don't understand what's going on.)

7- Conjugate the following verbs according to the given instructions:

a. Conjugate the verb "aprender" (to learn) in the present simple tense for "tú," "nosotros/nosotras," and "ustedes."

_____

_____

_____

b. Conjugate the verb "correr" (to run) in the progressive past tense for "yo," "él/ella/usted," and "ellos/ellas/ustedes."

_____

_____

_____

c. Conjugate the verb "escribir" (to write) in the progressive future tense for "tú," "vosotros/vosotras," and "ustedes."

_____

_____

_____

d. Conjugate the verb "hacer" (to do/make) in the future simple tense for "yo," "él/ella/usted," and "nosotros/nosotras."

_____

_____

_____

e. Conjugate the verb "decir" (to say) in the future simple tense for "tú," "nosotros/nosotras," and "ustedes."

_____

_____

_____

f. Conjugate the verb "tener" (to have) in the present simple tense for "yo," "vosotros/vosotras," and "ellos/ellas/ustedes."

_____

_____

_____

g. Conjugate the verb "poner" (to put/place) in the past simple for "tú," "nosotros/nosotras," and "ustedes."

_____

_____

_____

h. Conjugate the verb "venir" (to come) in the present simple tense for "yo," "nosotros/nosotras," and "ellos/ellas/ustedes."

_____

_____

_____

Answers:

a. Tú: aprendes
Nosotros/nosotras: aprendemos
Ustedes: aprenden

b. Yo: estuve corriendo
Él/ella/usted: estuvo corriendo
Ellos/ellas/ustedes: estuvieron corriendo

c. Tú: estarás escribiendo
Vosotros/vosotras: estareis escribiendo

Ustedes: estarán escribiendo

d. Yo: haré
Él/ella/usted: hará
Nosotros/nosotras: haremos

e. Tú: dirás
Nosotros/nosotras: diremos
Ustedes: dirán

f. Yo: tengo
Vosotros/vosotras: tenéis
Ellos/ellas/ustedes: tienen

g. Tú: pusiste
Nosotros/nosotras: pusimos
Ustedes: pusieron

h. Yo: vengo
Nosotros/nosotras: venimos
Ellos/ellas/ustedes: vienen

8- Translate the following sentences:

a. Me levanto temprano todas las mañanas y corro en el parque cercano.

———————————————————————

b. Los niños están jugando tranquilamente en la sala de estar.

_____

c. Ayer fui al supermercado y compré todos los ingredientes para preparar una cena deliciosa.

_____

d. Si llueve esta tarde, no podré ir al concierto que tanto esperaba.

_____

e. Mañana tendré una reunión importante en la oficina y tengo que preparar mi presentación.

_____

f. Durante las vacaciones de verano, viajaré por Europa y conoceré muchas ciudades nuevas.

_____

g. Hace años que no visito a mis abuelos, debería llamarlos para organizar un encuentro.

_____

h. No entiendo por qué mi jefe siempre está tan enojado, tal vez debería hablar con él para averiguar qué pasa.

_____

i. Me encanta la música clásica, siempre la escucho mientras trabajo en mi escritorio.

_____

j. Los estudiantes están estudiando arduamente para el examen final de la materia.

_____

k. Ayer recibí una carta de mi mejor amigo que vive en otro país, me hizo muy feliz leerla.

_____

l. Esta noche saldré a cenar con mi pareja a un restaurante nuevo que abrieron en el centro.

_____

m. Siempre trato de ser amable con las personas que conozco, creo que es importante tener una actitud positiva.

_____

n. En el parque hay muchas flores de colores diferentes, me encanta caminar por allí y admirarlas.

_____

o. Si gano la lotería, me compraré una casa en la playa y pasaré el resto de mi vida relajándome bajo el sol.

_____

Answers:

a. I wake up early every morning and run in the nearby park.

b. The children are playing quietly in the living room.

c. Yesterday I went to the supermarket and bought all the ingredients to prepare a delicious dinner.

d. If it rains this afternoon, I won't be able to go to the concert that I was looking forward to.

e. Tomorrow, I will have an important meeting at the office and I have to prepare my presentation.

f. During the summer vacation, I will travel around Europe and visit many new cities.

g. It's been years since I last visited my grandparents. I should call them to arrange a meeting.

h. I don't understand why my boss is always so angry. Maybe I should talk to him to find out what's going on.

i. I love classical music. I always listen to it while I work at my desk.

j. The students are studying hard for the final exam of the subject.

k. Yesterday, I received a letter from my best friend who lives in another country. It made me very happy to read it.

l. Tonight, I will go out to dinner with my partner at a new restaurant that opened downtown.

m. I always try to be kind to people I meet. I think it's important to have a positive attitude.

n. In the park there are many flowers of different colors, I love walking around and admiring them.

o. If I win the lottery, I will buy a house on the beach and spend the rest of my life relaxing under the sun.

SPANISH CULTURE AND CUSTOMS

Welcome to the last chapter of this book. You have explored the unknown lands of this wonderful language so far. As a last stop on our adventure, we will dive into the fascinating world of Spanish culture and customs. Understanding cultural differences is crucial to effectively communicating and building relationships with native speakers. So, let's get started!

Picture this: our protagonist, Sarah, traveled to Mexico to attend a funeral. She arrived wearing all black, as one does for a funeral, but to her surprise, everyone else was dressed casually and in colorful clothes. She immediately felt out of place and self-conscious. To make matters worse, when she was greeted by locals with two kisses, she had no idea what was going on. She felt embarrassed and wished she had done her research beforehand.

This scenario is a perfect example of why it's important to be aware of cultural customs when traveling or communicating with native speakers. It is time to explore some of the customs and traditions of Spanish-speaking countries, including greetings, holidays, and social norms. I will also provide you with valuable advice on how to immerse yourself in the culture and take away more from your experiences. So, let's jump in and learn how to navigate cultural contrasts like a pro!

SPANISH ACCENTS AND DIALECTS

First of all, let's talk about Spanish accents and dialects! Do you know how in English, there are different accents and even different vocabulary in different countries? Well, the same goes for Spanish. For example, if you go to Spain, you might find it challenging to understand someone from Andalusia if you're used to standard Castilian Spanish. The accent can be quite different, and some words may have different meanings depending on where you are. The grammar and even the intonation of sentences can vary depending on the region.

But don't worry, this doesn't mean that learning Spanish is difficult or pointless. Just like British people understand American people despite the differences in vocabulary and accent, Spanish speakers across the globe are aware of the differences and can still understand one another. Plus, learning the different accents and dialects can even make you more proficient in the language and give you a deeper understanding of Spanish culture. So, embrace the variety, and who knows, you might even find a new favorite accent.

While Spanish is the official language in more than 20 countries around the world, today we will take a closer look at some of the most representative ones. From the vibrant street markets of Colombia to the Spanish ham, each country has its own unique identity and charm.

Let's start with Mexico, a country that has captivated visitors with its delicious food, rich history, and colorful traditions. Mexicans are known for their warm hospitality and friendly nature, making it easy for visitors to feel at home. The country is also famous for its mariachi music and intricate Day of the Dead celebrations.

Colombia, on the other hand, boasts a diverse landscape of mountains, beaches, and rainforests. Colombians are passionate about their music and dance, with cumbia and salsa being popular genres. The country is also known for its coffee production and vibrant street art scene.

Moving north, the United States is home to a large Spanish-speaking population, particularly in states like California, Texas, and New Mexico. While each community has its unique cultural identity, they all share a love for spicy food, music, and traditions like the quinceañera and Día de los Muertos.

Argentina, famous for its delicious meat, premium football, and mate drink, is a country with a strong European influence. Argentinians are proud of their meat-based cuisine and love to socialize over a traditional asado (barbecue). The capital city of Buenos Aires is also a hub for arts and culture, with many theaters, museums, and galleries.

Spain, the birthplace of the Spanish language, is a country steeped in history and tradition. Spaniards are passionate about their food and wine, with each region having its own unique culinary specialties. Flamenco music and dance are also essential parts of the country's cultural heritage.

Peru, known for its ancient Incan ruins and stunning landscapes, is a country with a rich history and culture. Peruvians are proud of their culinary traditions, with dishes like ceviche and lomo saltado gaining popularity around the world. The country is also famous for its vibrant festivals and celebrations, like Inti Raymi and Carnaval de Cajamarca.

Venezuela, with its tropical beaches and vibrant nightlife, is a country with a strong Caribbean influence. Venezuelans are passionate about their music and dance, with genres like salsa and reggaeton being especially popular. The country is also known for its oil production and traditional crafts like hammock weaving.

Chile, a narrow strip of land on the western coast of South America, is a country with a diverse landscape that includes the Andes Mountains, the Atacama Desert, and, of course, the Pacific Ocean. Chileans are proud of their wine production and love to celebrate with traditional dishes like empanadas and pastel de choclo.

Ecuador, located on the equator, is a country with a rich biodiversity and cultural heritage. Ecuadorians are proud of their indigenous roots and celebrate them through traditional festivals and crafts like weaving and pottery. The country is also home to the stunning Galapagos Islands, which are famous for their unique wildlife.

Finally, Guatemala is a country with a strong Mayan heritage and a diverse landscape of volcanoes, lakes, and rainforests. Guatemalans are passionate about their traditional textiles and crafts, with many indigenous communities still practicing ancient techniques. The country is also known for its coffee production and vibrant celebrations like Semana Santa and Día de los Muertos.

HOW SPANISH-SPEAKING COUNTRIES VARY

Are you ready to spice up your Spanish? Well, one of the most intriguing things about the Spanish language is the incredible variety of accents and dialects that exist across the world. Just like in English, there are countless ways to say the same thing in Spanish. But don't worry, I'll guide you through some of the most famous ones!

First up, we have the Spanish accent, also known as Castilian Spanish. This is the standard accent used in Spain and is characterized by its crisp, clear pronunciation and its use of the "th" sound instead of the "s" sound for the letters "c" and "z." Some famous local words and expressions include:

- Vale (bah-leh): Okay
- Tío/Tía (tee-oh/tee-ah): Dude/girl
- Me mola (meh moh-lah): I like it
- Estar en el quinto pino (ehs-tahr ehn el keen-toh pee-noh): To be in the middle of nowhere

- Ponerse las botas (poh-nehr-seh lahs boh-tahs): To have a great meal

Next, we have the Mexican accent, which is perhaps the most well-known Spanish accent in the world due to Mexico's cultural influence. The Mexican accent is known for its singsong quality, with a rising intonation at the end of sentences. Some famous local words and expressions include:

- Chido (chee-doh): Cool
- Padre (pah-dreh): Awesome
- Chamba (chahm-bah): Job/work
- Qué onda (keh ohn-dah): What's up?
- Güey (wey): Dude

Moving on to South America, we have the Argentine accent, which is characterized by its distinct "sh" sound for the letters "ll" and "y." The Argentine accent is also known for its use of local slang and expressions. Some famous local words and expressions include:

- Che (cheh): Hey/dude
- Laburar (lah-boo-rahr): To work
- Bárbaro (bar-bah-roh): Great/awesome
- ¿Qué onda? (keh ohn-dah): What's up?
- Boludo/a (boh-loo-doh/boh-loo-dah): Fool/dude

In Colombia, we have the "paisa" accent, which is spoken in the Antioquia region and is known for its soft, melodious sound. Some famous local words and expressions include:

- Parcero/a (pahr-seh-roh/pahr-seh-rah): Friend/buddy
- Chimba (cheem-bah): Cool/awesome
- ¡Quihubo! (kee-oo-boh): What's up?
- Chévere (cheh-veh-reh): Great/cool
- Parche (pahr-cheh): Group of friends/hangout

For many of those who have learned neutral Spanish, the easiest Hispanic accent to identify, but the most difficult to learn, is Chilean. this accent is characterized by being very fast, sung, and closed, but it is also very fun and rhythmic! Some famous local words and expressions include:

- Pololo/a (poh-loh-loh/poh-loh-lah): Boyfriend/girlfriend
- Cachai (kah-chai): Do you understand?
- Bacán (bah-kan): Cool/awesome
- ¡Qué heavy! (keh heh-vee): That's tough/heavy
- Andar al lote (ahn-dahr ahl loh-teh): To be lost/confused

As you can see, the world of Spanish accents and dialects is rich and diverse, reflecting the unique cultural and linguistic traditions of each region. Whether you're learning Spanish for travel, business, or personal enrichment, taking the time to explore the different accents and expressions will deepen your understanding and appreciation of this beautiful language.

In conclusion, each Spanish-speaking country has its unique cultural identity and traditions. Whether you're exploring the bustling markets of Mexico or the stunning landscapes of Peru, there's always something new and exciting to discover.

TIPS ON NAVIGATING CULTURAL DIFFERENCES

As much as we love to travel and learn about new cultures, it's easy to unintentionally offend people when we don't understand their customs. But don't worry, with a little bit of knowledge and effort, you can avoid those uncomfortable situations. Let's go over some dos and don'ts when navigating cultural differences.

Dos:

- Research the culture before you go. This will help you understand the customs, values, and beliefs of the people you will be interacting with.
- Be respectful and open-minded. Show an interest in learning about the culture and be willing to adapt to their way of life.
- Learn some key phrases in their language. This will show that you are making an effort to communicate with them and they will appreciate it.
- Get familiar with greetings and formalities: In many Latin American countries, greetings and formalities are highly valued. Failing to greet someone properly, such as not saying "buenos días" (good morning) or "mucho gusto" (nice to meet you) when appropriate, can be seen as impolite or aloof.
- Dress appropriately. Some cultures have more conservative dress codes than others.
- Be aware of your body language. Gestures that are considered normal in your culture may be offensive to others.

Don'ts:

- Assume everyone speaks English. It's always a good idea to learn some basic words and phrases in the local language.
- Make assumptions about their culture based on stereotypes. Every culture is unique and diverse.
- Bring up politics or religion unless you know the person's point of view. These topics can be sensitive and should be approached with caution.
- Criticize their way of life or customs. Remember, you are a guest in their country.
- Be loud and obnoxious. Some cultures value quietness and restraint.
- Touch someone without permission. Personal space varies from culture to culture.

When it comes to Spanish culture, it's important to be aware of their history and traditions. While Catalonia and Franco may be fascinating topics to you, it's best to avoid discussing them unless you know the person's stance. And, as the majority of Latin Americans are Catholic, it's important to be respectful of their religion. By following these dos and don'ts, you can navigate cultural differences with confidence and respect. ¡Buen viaje!

GETTING GOOD AT CULTURAL IMMERSION

Are you planning to travel to Spain or Latin America soon? Well, it's not just about speaking the language fluently; it's also about immersing yourself in the culture. So, how do you become a master of cultural immersion? Fear not, I've got you covered!

First and foremost, try new foods! Spain is known for its culinary delights, so dive right in! Why not try cooking up some traditional dishes from Peru? Not only will your taste buds be grateful, but you'll also gain a deeper appreciation for the history and culture behind the food.

Next up, explore local customs. Argentina is famous for its tango dancing and mate drinking, so why not give it a try? By doing so, you'll acquire insight into the cultural values and traditions of the people.

Socializing with the locals is also a key component of cultural immersion. Take Bolivia, for example, where people are known for their hospitality and warmth. Strike up a conversation with a local and you might even make a new friend!

To really get a feel for the country, travel to different areas, even the lesser-known ones. Chile is a prime example, with its diverse landscapes ranging from deserts to glaciers. This way, you'll not only experience the beauty of the country but also learn about the history and culture of each region.

Attending live events is another great way to immerse yourself in the culture. In Colombia, for example, the Carnaval de Barranquilla is a must-see event that showcases the country's music, dance, and art.

Don't forget to keep up with the local news, as it will help you understand current events and trends. And if you're really serious about getting involved, why not volunteer with local communities or Spanish-speaking charities in your area? Not only will you be helping others, but you'll also be improving your language skills and gaining a deeper understanding of the culture. It's a win-win situation!

So, there you have it! By following these tips, you'll soon become a master of cultural immersion. Now, grab your passport, and let's go explore!

PRACTICE AND VOCABULARY

1- Read the following story about Álex and answer the questions below:

¿Te imaginas recorrer el continente americano en bicicleta? Pues Álex, un joven aventurero de Ohio, lo hizo posible. Empezando desde su ciudad natal, se adentró en una ruta emocionante hacia el sur de América, y en tan solo 24 meses conoció 11 países, ¡sí, leíste bien, 11 países!

Desde Panamá hasta Argentina, pasando por México, Honduras, Venezuela, Colombia, Brasil, Ecuador, Perú, Bolivia y Chile, Álex no dejó de maravillarse con cada lugar que visitaba. Los desiertos andinos y la fauna patagónica lo dejaron sin aliento, y no podemos culparlo, ¡es que son impresionantes!

Pero eso no es todo, el vasto mar peruano y las ruinas incas lo enamoraron aún más. Además, se aventuró a explorar la espesa selva amazónica de Colombia y a nadar en las aguas tropicales de Venezuela.

Y no solo aprendió a hablar español con fluidez, sino que también descubrió la cultura hispana de primera mano. Al volver a Ohio, se dio cuenta de que lo más valioso que había adquirido en su viaje no fue solo el idioma, sino la apreciación por todas las personas, los lugares, los sabores, los aromas y la música local.

Álex entendió que ese viaje lo había transformado en una persona mucho más tolerante y sencilla, capaz de disfrutar de las pequeñas cosas y valorar cada gesto auténtico. ¡Qué gran lección para todos nosotros!

Ahora mismo él sigue viviendo en su ciudad de origen, y está trabajando duro, pues tiene que ahorrar dinero para su próximo viaje por el mundo. El próximo destino será Japón. Por supuesto, allá no hablan español, asi que Alex tendrá que aprender un nuevo idioma.

¿Quién se anima a seguir los pasos de Álex y explorar el mundo con una mente abierta y un corazón aventurero?

Questions:

1. ¿De dónde es Álex? (Where is Alex from?)
2. ¿Por cuánto tiempo recorrió América del Sur en bicicleta? (For how long did he travel South America by bicycle?)
3. ¿Qué países visitó Álex en su viaje? (Which countries did Alex visit on his trip?)
4. ¿Qué paisajes naturales y sitios históricos visitó Álex durante su viaje? (What natural landscapes and historic sites did Alex visit during his trip?)
5. ¿Qué idioma aprendió Álex durante su viaje? (What language did Alex learn during his trip?)
6. ¿Cómo describirías la actitud de Álex hacia la cultura hispana después de su viaje? (How would you describe Alex's attitude towards Hispanic culture after his trip?)
7. ¿Cómo influyó el viaje de Álex en su personalidad y perspectiva de la vida? (How did Alex's trip influence his personality and perspective on life?)
8. ¿Cómo se sintió Álex al regresar a su hogar en Ohio después de su viaje? (How did Alex feel upon returning to his home in Ohio after his trip?)
9. ¿Dónde vive Alex actualmente y qué esta haciendo allí? ¿Por qué? (Where does Alex currently live and what is he doing there? Why?)
10. ¿Qué tendrá que hacer Alex en su próximo viaje? (What will Alex have to do on his next trip?)

Answers:

1. Álex es de Ohio. (Alex is from Ohio.)
2. Álex recorrió América del Sur en bicicleta durante 24 meses. (Alex traveled South America by bicycle for 24 months.)
3. Álex visitó Panamá, México, Honduras, Colombia, Venezuela, Brasil, Ecuador, Perú, Bolivia, Chile y Argentina en su viaje. (Alex visited Panama, Mexico, Honduras, Colombia, Venezuela, Brazil, Ecuador, Peru, Bolivia, Chile, and Argentina on his trip.)
4. Álex visitó una variedad de paisajes naturales como los desiertos andinos, la fauna patagónica, el vasto mar peruano, las ruinas incas, la selva amazónica de Colombia y las aguas tropicales de Venezuela. (Alex visited a variety of natural landscapes such as the Andean deserts, Patagonian fauna, the vast Peruvian sea, Incan ruins, the Colombian Amazon rainforest, and the tropical waters of Venezuela.)
5. Álex aprendió español durante su viaje. (Alex learned Spanish during his trip.)
6. Después de su viaje, Álex mostró una actitud de aprecio y disfrute hacia la cultura hispana. (After his trip, Alex showed an attitude of appreciation and enjoyment towards Hispanic culture.)
7. El viaje de Álex influyó en su personalidad haciéndolo más tolerante, simple y capaz de valorar las pequeñas cosas y los gestos auténticos. (Alex's trip influenced his personality, making him more tolerant, simple, and able to value the small things and authentic gestures.)

8. Álex se sintió cambiado y transformado después de su viaje, y se dio cuenta de que había ganado una perspectiva más amplia y apreciativa de la vida. (Alex felt changed and transformed after his trip, realizing that he had gained a broader and appreciative perspective on life.)

9. Álex vive en Ohio y está trabajando duro para ahorrar dinero para su próximo viaje. (Alex lives in Ohio and is working hard to save money for his next trip.)

10. Álex tendrá que aprender un nuevo idioma en Japón. (Alex will have to learn a new language in Japan.)

2- Write the name of the country whose dialect the following phrases belong to:

1. Vale tío, vamos a ponernos las botas en ese restaurante nuevo que me mola. (Okay man, let's get our boots on at that new restaurant that I love.)

_____

2. ¿Qué onda güey? La chamba está muy padre hoy. (What's up dude? The job is really awesome today.)

_____

3. ¡Bárbaro! Mañana voy a laburar desde casa, ¿qué onda con vos? (Great! Tomorrow I'm going to work from home, what's up with you?)

_____

4. ¡Quihubo parcero, que chimba que pudimos salir hoy en parche, estuvo chévere! (What's up friend, it was awesome that we could go out today with the group of friends, it was great!)

_____

5. Estuvimos en el quinto pino para llegar al concierto, pero valió la pena. (We were in the boondocks to get to the concert, but it was worth it.)

_____

6. Mi pololo es bacán y siempre me dice "cachai" cuando hablamos, aunque a veces me ando al lote y no le entiendo bien. (My boyfriend is cool and always says "do you understand?" when we talk, although sometimes I get lost and don't understand him well.)

_____

7. ¡Che boludo, qué onda! Vamos a laburar juntos hoy. (Hey dude, what's up! Let's work together today.)

———————————————

8. La música de esta fiesta está muy chida, güey. (The music at this party is very cool, dude.)

———————————————

Answers:

1. Spain
2. Mexico
3. Argentina
4. Colombia
5. Spain
6. Chile
7. Argentina
8. Mexico

Final advice and recommendations:

- Maximize the digital world and available Spanish to improve your language skills.
- Read online Spanish newspapers like El País, 8 Columnas, and El Diario.
- Switch the language of your favorite TV series to Spanish, choosing one with everyday language rather than technical vocabulary. *Friends* is a great option!
- Order in Spanish at your favorite Spanish restaurant and use the language as much as possible.

- Join Spanish language exchange groups on social media or apps like Tandem or HelloTalk to practice with native speakers.

The more you expose yourself to the language, the more you'll improve. Enjoy this whole new world you just discovered ¡Buena suerte, y hasta pronto!

BONUS: THE ULTIMATE SECRET TO MASTERING SPANISH PRONUNCIATION

L earning to speak Spanish fluently is a great accomplishment for anyone who wishes to expand their cultural horizons and connect with millions of people around the world. However, for many English speakers, mastering Spanish pronunciation is a daunting challenge. In this bonus section, I will provide you with a comprehensive guide to help you achieve perfect pronunciation for your Spanish.

As we already learned in the first chapter, Spanish and English share many consonant sounds, but there are five sounds that are always hard for English speakers to master. Let me briefly remind you of them:

1. **The letter "h"**: This one is always silent, which can be confusing for English speakers who are used to pronouncing it. For example, the word "hola" is pronounced as "ola" in Spanish.

2. **The letter "j":** Its sound is similar to the "h" sound in English, but it is pronounced further back in the throat. To produce the sound, try saying the English "h" sound while exhaling sharply, like a mad cat. For example, the word "joven" is pronounced as "ho-ven" in Spanish.

3. **The letter "ñ":** The "ñ" is a whole new world for non-native Spanish speakers since its sound does not exist in English, and can be difficult for English speakers to master. To produce the sound, try saying English words like "canyon." The sound made up by the "ny" is quite similar to the Spanish "ñ." For example, the word "niño" is pronounced as "nee-nyo" in Spanish.

4. **The letters "ll" and "y":** As I mentioned only briefly in the first chapter, in some Spanish-speaking countries, the "ll" sound is pronounced as a "y" sound, while in others they are pronounced as a "sh" sound. Nevertheless, you will have to choose a unique Spanish accent to learn their proper pronunciation. Yet, I will remind you of the sound for "ll" and "y" in neutral Spanish. So, to produce this sound, just do it in the same way you would pronounce "y" in English; For example, the word "lluvia" (rain) is pronounced as "you-via" in Spanish. In the same way, "yema" (bud) is pronounced (yeh-mah).

5. **The letter "r":** In Spanish, the "r" is pronounced with a single tap or flap of the tongue against the roof of the mouth, just behind the front teeth. This is called an alveolar flap or trill, and it produces a distinctive rolling sound. For example, "perro" (dog) is pronounced as "peh-rro" with a trilled "r" sound. In English, the sound of the letter "r" is much softer.

Think of the word "pearl" or "ride"; the tip of your tongue never touches the palate, therefore the characteristic vibration of the rolling "r" of Spanish is not produced.

Moving forward, Spanish vowels are relatively easy to pronounce, but some differences between English and Spanish vowel sounds can certainly confuse you. Here are some tips for getting the Spanish vowel sounds right:

1. **The letter "a":** This vowel is always pronounced as "ah," as in "father." For example, the word "casa" is pronounced as "cah-sa."
2. **The letter "e":** It's pronounced as "eh," as in "let." For example, the word "mesa" is pronounced as "meh-sa."
3. **The letter "i":** Must be pronounced as "ee," as in "meet." For example, the word "hijo" is pronounced as "ee-ho" in Spanish.
4. **The letter "o":** This one sounds like the "o" in the English word "go." For example, the word "hola" is pronounced "oh-la."
5. **The letter "u":** Must be pronounced like the "oo" in "moon." For example, the word "uno" is pronounced "oo-no." This vowel is particularly difficult for English speakers because its Spanish sound does not exist in English. That is, there is a similar sound—like the "oo" in "moon"—but it is not the same. While in English the sound "oo" comes from the throat, in Spanish it is achieved by bringing the lips forward and slightly squeezing them, leaving a small space to let the air out of

the mouth—similar to how we would do it when whistling or giving a kiss.

Spanish pronunciation is relatively simple and straightforward compared to many other languages. Unlike many languages where spelling and pronunciation are not always consistent, Spanish is a phonetic language, meaning that words are pronounced as they are written. This is a major advantage for language learners and the ultimate secret to mastering Spanish pronunciation I promised you: **Once you master the sounds of each letter of the Spanish alphabet, you will be able to read and pronounce all the words in Spanish correctly.**

One of the primary reasons for this is that Spanish has a relatively small number of phonemes (distinct sounds), making it easier to learn than languages with larger phonemic inventories. In contrast, picture this: Mandarin Chinese has about 420 sounds, including consonants, vowels, and diphthongs (Encyclopedia Britannica., n.d.).

In Spanish, there are only five vowel sounds, while in English, there are more than ten. Additionally, Spanish has fewer consonant sounds than English, which further simplifies the language.

Another factor that makes Spanish pronunciation easier to master is that many of the sounds in Spanish are similar to those in English. For example, the Spanish "b" and "v" sounds are identical or very similar to the English "b" sound.

One of the biggest fears that language learners have is not sounding like a native speaker. And this applies to all people who speak a second language, not just to Spanish amateurs. While it's certainly true that mastering a foreign language's pronunciation takes time and practice, it's also important to remember that having an accent is not necessarily a bad thing.

Accents are a natural part of language diversity, and they reflect a person's unique background and linguistic history.

Moreover, learning a new language is an achievement in itself, regardless of whether you sound like a native speaker or not. The goal of language learning should be effective communication, not necessarily achieving native-like fluency. It's worth remembering that most native Spanish speakers will be impressed that you've made the effort to learn their language, regardless of whether you have an accent or not.

It's important to embrace your accent and make it part of your linguistic identity. It can be a nice or distinctive trait rather than a liability, as it can make you stand out and add to the diversity of the communities you're part of. So, don't be discouraged by the prospect of not sounding like a native speaker; embrace your unique voice and celebrate your love for the Spanish language!

BONUS: PRACTICE AND VOCABULARY

1- Learn new tenses to expand your knowledge of Spanish to the highest level. Observe the explanation and its examples.

a. Preterite Perfect and Imperfect:

In Spanish, the preterite perfect (also known as past simple) and imperfect are both past tenses, but they have different uses. The preterite perfect is used to describe completed actions in the recent past, while the imperfect is used to describe ongoing or habitual actions in the past.

Here is a table with the conjugations in all the grammatical persons of 10 verbs in the preterit perfect or past simple tense in Spanish:

Verbo	Yo	Tú	Él/ Ella/ Usted	Nosotros/ Nosotras	Vosotros/ Vosotras	Ellos/ Ellas/ Ustedes
Salir	Salí	Saliste	Salió	Salimos	Salisteis	Salieron
Escapar	Escapé	Escapaste	Escapó	Escapamos	Escapasteis	Escaparon
Comer	Comí	Comiste	Comió	Comimos	Comisteis	Comieron
Hablar	Hablé	Hablaste	Habló	Hablamos	Hablasteis	Hablaron
Caminar	Caminé	Caminaste	Caminó	Caminamos	Caminasteis	Caminaron
Correr	Corrí	Corriste	Corrió	Corrimos	Corristeis	Corrieron
Vivir	Viví	Viviste	Vivió	Vivimos	Vivisteis	Vivieron
Llegar	Llegué	Llegaste	Llegó	Llegamos	Llegasteis	Llegaron
Tomar	Tomé	Tomaste	Tomó	Tomamos	Tomasteis	Tomaron
Cantar	Canté	Cantaste	Cantó	Cantamos	Cantasteis	Cantaron

For example:

- Después de que ella terminó de estudiar, se fue a la cama. (After she finished studying, she went to bed.)

- Cuando él recibió la noticia, sintió una gran alegría. (When he received the news, he felt a great joy.)
- A pesar de que llovió todo el día, disfrutamos de nuestras vacaciones. (Although it rained all day, we enjoyed our vacation.)
- Tan pronto como ellos llegaron a la playa, se quitaron los zapatos. (As soon as they arrived at the beach, they took off their shoes.)
- Una vez que terminaron de cocinar, comenzaron a preparar la mesa. (Once they finished cooking, they started setting the table.)

Now, I present the same list but with these conjugated verbs in the imperfect past tense of Spanish:

Verbo	Yo	Tú	Él/ Ella/ Usted	Nosotros/ Nosotras	Vosotro/ Vosotras	Ellos/ Ellas/ Ustedes
Salir	Salía	Salías	Salía	Salíamos	Salíais	Salían
Escapar	Escapaba	Escapabas	Escapaba	Escapábamos	Escapabais	Escapaban
Comer	Comía	Comías	Comía	Comíamos	Comíais	Comían
Hablar	Hablaba	Hablabas	Hablaba	Hablábamos	Hablabais	Hablaban
Caminar	Caminaba	Caminabas	Caminaba	Caminábamos	Caminabais	Caminaban
Correr	Corría	Corrías	Corría	Corríamos	Corríais	Corrían
Vivir	Vivía	Vivías	Vivía	Vivíamos	Vivíais	Vivían
Llegar	Llegaba	Llegabas	Llegaba	Llegábamos	Llegabais	Llegaban
Tomar	Tomaba	Tomabas	Tomaba	Tomábamos	Tomabais	Tomaban
Cantar	Cantaba	Cantabas	Cantaba	Cantábamos	Cantabais	Cantaban

For example:

- Cuando era niño, siempre jugaba al fútbol con mis amigos del barrio. (When I was a child, I always used to play soccer with my friends from the neighborhood.)
- Mientras estudiábamos para el examen, nos dimos cuenta de que nos faltaba un libro importante. (While we were studying for the exam, we realized that we were missing an important book.)
- A pesar de que llovía, la gente seguía haciendo compras en el mercado. (Despite the fact that it was raining, people kept shopping at the market.)
- Cuando vivía en Nueva York, iba al cine todos los fines de semana. (When I lived in New York, I used to go to the movies every weekend.)
- Mientras preparábamos la cena, escuchábamos música en la radio. (While we were preparing dinner, we were listening to music on the radio.)

b. Future Conditional:

The future conditional in Spanish is a tense that is used to talk about hypothetical actions that could happen in the future, but that depend on a previous condition. For example, in the sentence "Si tuviera más dinero, viajaría por todo el mundo" (If I had more money, I would travel around the world), the verb "viajaría" (I would travel) is in the future conditional, since it indicates a hypothetical action that would only occur if the condition of having more money is met.

The future conditional can also be used to express a wish or a request in a more polite way. For example, in the sentence "I would like to go to the movies tonight," the verb "would like" is in the future conditional and is used to express a wish in a more polite way.

Here is a table with the conjugations in all the grammatical persons in some future conditional verbs in Spanish:

Verbo	Yo	Tú	Él/Ella/Usted	Nosotros/Nosotras	Vosotro/Vosotras	Ellos/Ellas/Ustedes
Tener	Tendría	Tendrías	Tendría	Tendríamos	Tendríais	Tendrían
Poder	Podría	Podrías	Podría	Podríamos	Podríais	Podrían
Saber	Sabría	Sabrías	Sabría	Sabríamos	Sabríais	Sabrían
Querer	Querría	Querrías	Querría	Querríamos	Querríais	Querrían
Hacer	Haría	Harías	Haría	Haríamos	Haríais	Harían
Decir	Diría	Dirías	Diría	Diríamos	Diríais	Dirían
Ir	Iría	Irías	Iría	Iríamos	Iríais	Irían
Venir	Vendría	Vendrías	Vendría	Vendríamos	Vendríais	Vendrían
Ser	Sería	Serías	Sería	Seríamos	Seríais	Serían
Estar	Estaría	Estarías	Estaría	Estaríamos	Estaríais	Estarían

Examples:

- Si tuviera más tiempo, me gustaría aprender a tocar el piano. (If I had more time, I would like to learn how to play the piano.)
- Si pudiera hablar francés, viajaría a París sin dudarlo. (If I could speak French, I would travel to Paris without hesitation.)
- Si supiera la respuesta, te ayudaría con el problema. (If I knew the answer, I would help you with the problem.)
- Si quisieras venir conmigo, te mostraría mi ciudad favorita. (If you wanted to come with me, I would show you my favorite city.)
- Si fuera millonario, donaría una parte de mi dinero a obras benéficas. (If I were a millionaire, I would donate a portion of my money to charitable causes.)

2- Put these new tenses into practice:

a. Write a short biography of a famous person in Spanish, using the past perfect or simple tense to talk about their achievements and important events in their life.

For example: Julio César **fue** un político romano. **Nació** en Roma, **creció** y **estudió** allí hasta que **cumplió** la mayoría de edad... (Julius Caesar was a Roman politician. He was born in Rome, grew up and studied there until he came of age...)

_____

_____

_____

_____

_____

_____

_____

_____

b. Complete the following sentences with the correct form of the past perfect (or simple) of the verb in parentheses:

1. Yo _____ (comprar) un regalo para mi mamá.
2. Ellos _____ (viajar) por Europa el verano pasado.
3. Tú _____ (estudiar) mucho para el examen.
4. Él _____ (escribir) una novela el año pasado.
5. Nosotros _____ (aprender) a tocar la guitarra en el conservatorio.
6. Vosotros _____ (hacer) una cena deliciosa para vuestros amigos.
7. Ella _____ (visitar) a su familia en Navidad.
8. Ustedes _____ (ver) la película en el cine anoche.

Answers:

1. compré
2. viajaron
3. estudiaste
4. escribió
5. aprendimos
6. hicísteis
7. visitó
8. vieron

c. Create a story in which you use the imperfect tense to describe the scenes, characters, and actions that occurred.

For example: **Había** una vez un león llamado Magnus. Él **estaba** muy hambriento y **esperaba** tras un arbusto por su presa... (Once upon a time there was a lion named Magnus. He was very hungry and waited behind a bush for his prey...)

_____

_____

_____

_____

_____

_____

_____

d. Write a list of 10 things you would do if you had an extra day off. Use the conditional to describe the activities you would like to do.

For example: Si no **tuviera** que trabajar el domingo, **iría** a conocer el nuevo acuario de la ciudad. (If I didn't have to work on Sunday, I'd go to see the new aquarium in town.)

1. _____
2. _____
3. _____
4. _____
5. _____
6. _____
7. _____
8. _____
9. _____

CONCLUSION

Learning a new language is a journey that requires dedication, effort, and patience. I commend you for committing yourself to this adventure, and for taking the time to invest in your personal development. Learning Spanish—like any other new language—will open up doors to new opportunities, whether it be for travel, work, and, who knows, maybe love—as was my case!

We started this journey together by discussing the benefits of learning Spanish, including the ability to communicate with millions of people all over the world. The first chapter of this book focused on the Spanish alphabet and pronunciation. I have provided a guide to the sounds and letters of the Spanish language, as well as tips and tricks for mastering the pronunciation, funny useful exercises and vocabulary lists to help you practice and build your skills at the bottom of every chapter.

Chapter 2 focused on essential Spanish vocabulary. We covered keywords and phrases that you're likely to encounter in everyday conversations that will allow you to describe objects, housework, name animals, professions, and hobbies, among other things.

Later, in Chapter 3, we turned our attention to numbers and time. We covered how to tell time in Spanish, as well as how to count and use numbers in various contexts.

In Chapter 4, we focused on common words and phrases for everyday situations. We addressed topics such as greetings and introductions, ordering food at a restaurant, expressing likes and dislikes, and making small talk.

Chapter 5 delved into Spanish grammar. We covered important grammatical concepts such as gender, singular and plural forms, and sentence structure.

Moving on to Chapter 6, we emphasized the importance of verbs in Spanish. We learned how to conjugate regular and irregular verbs, as well as how to use verbs in different tenses.

The last chapter focused on Spanish culture and customs. It brought you an overview of the rich history and traditions of the Spanish-speaking world, as well as tips and insights for navigating cultural differences. I told you an exciting story about a bike traveler that I strongly encourage you to read over and over again.

Finally, in the Bonus chapter, I shared with you the ultimate secret to mastering Spanish pronunciation by showing you additional tips and exercises to help you fine-tune your pronunciation and build your confidence in speaking Spanish. By the end, we also talked about the importance of not being ashamed of our foreign accent when speaking Spanish or any other second language, since it is nothing more than part of our identity.

It is necessary to reinforce what you have learned so far so that it sticks in your memory. Remember to use multiple learning techniques such as flashcards, recording your own voice, making mind maps, labeling items in your home, and speaking to yourself in the mirror. Immerse yourself in Spanish-speaking environments, listen to Spanish music and watch Spanish films, and engage in conversations with native speakers. The more you expose yourself to the language, the more comfortable and confident you will become. These techniques may seem silly at first, but they are proven to be effective in reinforcing learning and retaining information.

I want to take this opportunity to share my own success story with you. As a native Spanish speaker who had to learn English, I can confidently say that learning a new language can be challenging but also incredibly rewarding. By having English and Spanish as my skill sets, I have been able to travel to so many countries in the world, and have meaningful, interesting conversations with people from different backgrounds. Learning Spanish will open doors to new opportunities and experiences that may have otherwise been unavailable.

As we conclude, I encourage you to take the next steps in your language-learning journey. Incorporate Spanish into your daily life by thinking in Spanish, using Spanish words to navigate your surroundings, and practicing your speaking skills whenever possible. Remember that the more you immerse yourself in the language, the faster you will pick it up.

I would love to read your feedback on this book and how it has helped you in your language-learning journey. Reviews are an important way to share your opinions and experiences to help others who are also interested in learning Spanish. **By leaving a review, you will inspire and encourage others to take the leap and start speaking Spanish themselves.**

Scan the QR Code to leave a review!

Learn Spanish for Adult Beginners: Speak Confidently & Impress Your Amigos has been a comprehensive guide aimed at providing you with everything you need to quickly learn Spanish. If you continue to follow the tips and exercises provided in each chapter, you will undoubtedly build your skills and confidence in speaking and understanding Spanish. I hope that this book has been a valuable resource for you and that it has inspired you to continue learning and exploring the rich and vibrant world of the Spanish language and culture.

¡Gracias y hasta pronto!

REFERENCES

Az Quotes. (n.d.). *Angela Carter quote.* A-Z Quotes. https://www.azquotes.com/
  quote/611535

Encyclopedia Britannica. (n.d.). *Chinese languages.* https://www.britannica.com/
  topic/Chinese-languages

Newsdle. (n.d.). *Brief history of Spanish language.* https://www.newsdle.com/
  blog/brief-history-of-spanish-language#:~:text=Spanish%20originated%
  20in%20the%20Iberian,spread%20around%20the%20world%20thereafter.

Tell Me In Spanish. (n.d.). *Spanish language statistics.* https://www.tellmeinspan
  ish.com/stats/spanish-language-statistics/

WhyNotSpanish. (2018). *¡Ojalá! The Spanish word with Arabic origins.* https://
  www.whynotspanish.com/ojala-spanish-word-arabic-origins/

BOOK 2: MEDICAL SPANISH FOR HEALTHCARE HEROES

MEDICAL SPANISH FOR HEALTHCARE HEROES

A COMPREHENSIVE GUIDE TO QUICKLY MASTER
VITAL TERMINOLOGY, EXPERTLY NAVIGATE MEDICAL
INTERACTIONS AND DELIVER SUPERIOR PATIENT
CARE IN 31 DAYS!

SOL MANCILLA

INTRODUCTION

The more I understood the patient's story, the more I realized that it was not just the disease that was important; it was the patient's story that needed to be understood.

— BERNARD LOWN

Picture this: Within the bustling environment of a hospital, a dedicated healthcare professional stands at the bedside of a patient. In this critical moment, they share more than just a room; they share an unspoken connection built on trust and understanding. This connection transcends mere medical knowledge—it's about empathy, reassurance, and effective communication. Yet, in this scenario, there's a challenging obstacle, a barrier that often separates this profound connection: a language barrier. The patient, speaking Spanish, yearns for comfort and clarity, while the healthcare professional strives to provide the best care possible, hindered by linguistic limitations. This is not just a hypothetical scene; it's a reality faced by countless healthcare heroes every day.

You may agree with me on something: Communication is not a trivial skill; it allows people to establish and strengthen conventions, bonds, and agreements on which our entire social dynamic and our civilization are built.

In a medical context, communication goes beyond symbols: It's a lifeline, a conduit through which expertise and compassion flow. Language barriers are undesirable challenges in this context. If the patient is not able to properly communicate their affairs to the medical professional and vice versa, the consequences are profound. The need for effective transmission in healthcare, especially in culturally diverse societies, is not a matter of mere convenience; it's an imperative.

Consider this startling fact: Spanish is the second most spoken language in the United States, with over 40 million native speakers and millions more who are bilingual (Thompson, 2021). Yet, a significant portion of healthcare professionals find themselves navigating the complex topography of patient care without the linguistic tools required to provide optimal care to Spanish-speaking patients. This discrepancy leads to misunderstandings, misdiagnoses, and a profound lack of trust in the healthcare system, and ultimately can potentially affect people's health and well-being. It's a challenge that has far-reaching implications, touching the lives of countless individuals who seek healthcare.

Allow me to introduce myself. I am an advocate for communication. I am just an observer of the healthcare system who believes unequivocally in the power and importance of human communication. Through my own experience and that of people in my surroundings, I have noticed the frustrations and limitations that healthcare professionals face when they cannot effectively communicate with their patients.

In many cases within this sector, healthcare professionals work alongside interpreters to bridge the language gap between them and their patients. While this approach ensures understanding, there is immense value in healthcare providers being able to communicate directly with their patients and their families. The ability to speak in Spanish empowers nurses, doctors, and other professionals, instilling a sense of competence and fostering a deeper and more human connection with those in their care.

As a bilingual native Spanish speaker with a career in communication, I have dedicated my life to finding solutions to different challenges related to language barriers. I understand the significance of compassionate care, and I firmly believe that language should never impede it. That's why I am writing this book—to empower healthcare professionals like you with the tools to break down language barriers, foster understanding, and provide the highest level of care to every patient, regardless of the language they speak.

This book possesses a clear and unwavering purpose: to boost healthcare professionals' communication skills and to help them learn Spanish not merely as a language but as an indispensable means of enhancing the quality of care they offer to Spanish-speaking patients. It is about bridging the gap between the mastery of medical terminology and the ability to engage in meaningful conversations with patients, their families, and the broader community.

These pages are more than just a language guide; they contain a comprehensive resource that is meticulously crafted to transform healthcare professionals into confident and effective communicators in Spanish.

This guide is divided into seven chapters, each thoughtfully structured to provide you with the knowledge and skills necessary for success.

Throughout the book, you will find pronunciation guides and phonetic support to ensure that your spoken Spanish is clear and confident. The content is structured for easy navigation, and practical exercises make learning engaging and effective.

I extend an invitation to venture on this exceptional trip to learn Spanish for healthcare. Irrespective of your current level of Spanish proficiency, this book will equip you with tools to enhance your communication with Spanish-speaking patients. It will empower you in your healthcare career, enabling you to provide compassionate, efficient care to a broader and more diverse patient population.

As you turn the pages of this book, you take the first deliberate step towards breaking down language barriers in healthcare. I ask you to seize this opportunity, to dive into the first chapter, and to commit wholeheartedly to becoming a healthcare hero who communicates with efficacy, empathizes profoundly, and cares comprehensively.

Turn the page; your journey commences now. *¡Adelante!*

BUILDING THE BRIDGE: BASICS OF SPANISH FOR HEALTHCARE

For healthcare professionals, effective communication is a—literally—vital skill. The ability to convey critical information, understand patients' needs, and provide clear instructions can be a matter of life and death. Now, imagine encountering a patient who speaks Spanish as their primary language, and you, as a healthcare professional, find yourself grappling with the language barrier. This is where our journey begins.

This first chapter is your launching pad into the realm of Spanish for healthcare. I admit that you have a demanding profession, with little time to spare for elaborate language courses. That's why this whole book is designed to be precise, focused, and tailored to the unique demands of your field.

Through the following pages, we will lay the foundation of your Spanish language skills, equipping you with the rudimentary grammar, critical vocabulary, and correct pronunciation necessary to navigate healthcare contexts with confidence and competence.

We'll start with the understanding that Spanish is a doorway to deeper, more human connections with your patients. It's about building trust, ensuring accurate diagnoses, and delivering care with empathy. You are now embarking on a journey to break down language barriers, provide superior care to Spanish-speaking patients, and enhance your professional profile in the healthcare domain.

¡Comencemos!

MORE THAN JUST A LANGUAGE

With approximately 460 million native speakers, Spanish holds the distinguished title of being the second most spoken language in the world, trailing only behind Mandarin Chinese (McCarthy, 2020). It's a testament to the rich diversity of cultures and communities it connects. Yet, its significance in the healthcare landscape extends far beyond sheer numbers.

Let's zoom in on the United States, where the Spanish language finds a thriving home. According to the Instituto Cervantes (Martinez, 2015), a renowned institution dedicated to the Spanish language and culture, the United States boasts the second-highest concentration of Spanish speakers on the planet, surpassed only by Mexico. This fact paints a compelling picture: A substantial portion of patients navigating the American health-care system converse primarily in Spanish. This demographic reality serves as a poignant reminder of the importance of Spanish proficiency for healthcare professionals.

However, the essence of learning this beautiful language in the healthcare arena goes beyond a mere statistical imperative. It's a journey that transcends numbers and charts, aiming to bridge a profound communication gap. Think of it this way: Learning Spanish isn't just about adding a language skill to your resume; it's about dismantling barriers that separate patients from their caregivers.

Consider the role of interpreters, those professionals who facilitate communication between patients and healthcare providers. While their assistance is undeniably practical, it can inadvertently create a sense of automation and detachment in the patient–professional relationship. Conversations become transactional, as clinical information is relayed through an intermediary.

Now, imagine the transformation that occurs when healthcare professionals can converse directly with their patients in their native language. It's like opening a window into their world, allowing you to connect on a deeper level. It's not just about relaying medical information; it's about forging a connection built on empathy, understanding, and trust. It's about giving autonomy to healthcare professionals in the field to engage in meaningful conversations that transcend clinical verbiage.

As a healthcare professional, your commitment to patient care extends beyond the clinical aspects. It encompasses the emotional and psychological well-being of your patients. The ability to converse with them in their preferred language is a powerful gesture of respect, a demonstration of empathy, and a catalyst for building trust. It empowers you to truly understand your patients' needs, fears, and aspirations, leading to more effective diagnoses and treatments.

The pages that follow will equip you with the tools and knowledge needed to bridge this language intermission and elevate your healthcare practice to new heights.

BASIC SPANISH GRAMMAR

One of the key characteristics that set Spanish apart is its phonetic nature. It means that words are pronounced precisely as they are written. Unlike some other languages where pronunciation can be a labyrinth of exceptions, in Spanish, what you see is what you say. This phonetic quality lends a sense of predictability and consistency to the language, making it more approachable for learners.

Now, let's bridge this language knowledge to your healthcare practice. Imagine being able to construct simple sentences in Spanish. It's akin to unlocking a treasure trove of understanding when it comes to your patient's symptoms and medical procedures. The ability to communicate basic concepts can be a game-changer in patient interactions.

For instance, consider the significance of being able to ask a simple question like *¿Dónde le duele?* (Where does it hurt?). This straightforward inquiry can provide invaluable insights into a patient's condition, enabling you to pinpoint the source of discomfort and take swift action.

Likewise, the power of being able to make statements such as *Necesito tomar su presión arterial* (I need to take your blood pressure) should not be underestimated. This concise sentence not only conveys your intention but also reassures the patient by keeping them informed about the procedure. It's a bridge between medical expertise and patient understanding.

These examples illustrate how even a basic grasp of Spanish grammar can significantly enhance patient interactions in healthcare settings. It's about breaking down the language barrier, one sentence at a time, and forging connections that transcend linguistic differences. In the subsequent sections of this chapter, we will delve deeper into the foundations of Spanish grammar, equipping you with the tools to construct meaningful sentences and engage in more effective patient communication.

Let's dive into the foundations of Spanish grammar one by one.

Subject Pronouns

Subject pronouns are essential elements in constructing sentences as they indicate who or what is performing the action of the verb. Here are the Spanish subject pronouns along with their English translations:

Subject pronouns (*pronombres personales*)	English translation
Yo	I
Tú	You: informal singular
Él / Ella	He / She
Usted	You: formal singular
Nosotros / Nosotras	We
Vosotros / Vosotras	You all: informal plural
Ellos (masculine) / Ellas (feminine)	They
Ustedes	You all: formal plural

Examples:

- *Yo hablo español* (I speak Spanish)
- *Tú estudias medicina* (You study medicine)
- *Él es el médico* (He is the doctor)
- *Nosotros trabajamos en el hospital* (We work at the hospital)

Masculine and Feminine Nouns

In Spanish, nouns have gender, which can be masculine (*masculino*) or feminine (*femenino*). Additionally, articles must match the gender and number of nouns. Here's a chart with some examples:

Gender	Noun	Article	English translation
Masculine	El chico	El (The)	The boy
	El hospital	El (The)	The hospital
	Los libros	Los (The)	The books
	Los estudiantes	Los (The)	The students
Feminine	La chica	La (The)	The girl
	La enfermera	La (The)	The nurse
	Las flores	Las (The)	The flowers
	Las amigas	Las (The)	The friends (all female)

Verb Conjugations

Spanish verbs undergo conjugation to match the subject of the sentence in terms of person and number. Let's examine the present simple, past simple, and future simple tenses, using the basic verbs ser, estar, and tener.

In the following chart, you'll find the conjugation in the **present simple** tense for the verbs ser (to be), estar (to be), and tener (to have).

Ser (to be [for permanent states]):

Subject pronouns	Conjugation	English translation
Yo	soy	I am
Tú	eres	You are (informal singular)
Él / Ella / Usted	es	He / She / You (formal) is/ are
Nosotros / Nosotras	somos	We are
Vosotros / Vosotras	sois	You all are (informal plural)
Ellos / Ellas / Ustedes	son	They / You all (formal) are

Estar (to be [for temporary states]):

Subject pronouns	Conjugation	English translation
Yo	estoy	I am
Tú	estás	You are (informal singular)
Él / Ella / Usted	está	He / She / You (formal) is/ are
Nosotros / Nosotras	estamos	We are
Vosotros / Vosotras	estáis	You all are (informal plural)
Ellos / Ellas / Ustedes	están	They / You all (formal) are

Tener (to have):

Subject pronouns	Conjugation	English translation
Yo	tengo	I have
Tú	tienes	You have (informal singular)
Él / Ella / Usted	tiene	He / She / You (formal) has/ have
Nosotros / Nosotras	tenemos	We have
Vosotros / Vosotras	tenéis	You all have (informal plural)
Ellos / Ellas / Ustedes	tienen	They / You all (formal) have

Now, let's take a look at the conjugation for these verbs in the **past simple** form.

Ser (to be):

Subject pronouns	Conjugation	English translation
Yo	fui	I was
Tú	fuiste	You were (informal singular)
Él / Ella / Usted	fue	He / She / You (formal) was/ were
Nosotros / Nosotras	fuimos	We were
Vosotros / Vosotras	fuisteis	You all were (informal plural)
Ellos / Ellas / Ustedes	fueron	They / You all (formal) were

Estar (to be):

Subject pronouns	Conjugation	English translation
Yo	estuve	I was
Tú	estuviste	You were (informal singular)
Él / Ella / Usted	estuvo	He / She / You (formal) was/ were
Nosotros / Nosotras	estuvimos	We were
Vosotros / Vosotras	estuvisteis	You all were (informal plural)
Ellos / Ellas / Ustedes	estuvieron	They / You all (formal) were

Tener (to have):

Subject pronouns	Conjugation	English translation
Yo	tuve	I had
Tú	tuviste	You had (informal singular)
Él / Ella / Usted	tuvo	He / She / You (formal) had
Nosotros / Nosotras	tuvimos	We had
Vosotros / Vosotras	tuvisteis	You all had (informal plural)
Ellos / Ellas / Ustedes	tuvieron	They / You all (formal) had

For **future simple:**

Ser (to be):

Subject pronouns	Conjugation	English translation
Yo	seré	I will be
Tú	serás	You will be (informal singular)
Él / Ella / Usted	será	He / She / You (formal) will be
Nosotros / Nosotras	seremos	We will be
Vosotros / Vosotras	seréis	You all will be (informal plural)
Ellos / Ellas / Ustedes	serán	They / You all (formal) will be

Estar (to be):

Subject pronouns	Conjugation	English translation
Yo	estaré	I will be
Tú	estarás	You will be (informal singular)
Él / Ella / Usted	estará	He / She / You (formal) will be
Nosotros / Nosotras	estaremos	We will be
Vosotros / Vosotras	estaréis	You all will be (informal plural)
Ellos / Ellas / Ustedes	estarán	They / You all (formal) will be

Tener (to have):

Subject pronouns	Conjugation	English translation
Yo	*tendré*	I will have
Tú	*tendrás*	You will have (informal singular)
Él / Ella / Usted	*tendrá*	He / She / You (formal) will have
Nosotros / Nosotras	*tendremos*	We will have
Vosotros / Vosotras	*tendréis*	You all will have (informal plural)
Ellos / Ellas / Ustedes	*tendrán*	They / You all (formal) will have

Basic Sentence Structure

While Spanish and English share some similarities in sentence structure, there are also notable differences.

In both Spanish and English, the basic sentence structure follows the subject-verb-object (SVO) order, where

- **Subject (S)** refers to the person or thing performing the action.
- **Verb (V)** represents the action being performed.
- **Object (O)** is the receiver of the action.

Let me illustrate this similarity with the following example:

- *Ella (S) lee (V) un libro (O)* (She [S] reads [V] a book [O]).
  This sentence has SVO structure in both languages.

However, there are still myriad differences from the English structure:

- **Adjective placement:** In Spanish, adjectives typically follow the noun they describe. This is different from English, where adjectives often precede the noun. For example, in Spanish, you would say "Una flor hermosa" (A beautiful flower), where "*flor*" is the object and "*hermosa*" is the adjective.
- **Subject pronouns:** While English often includes subject pronouns (I, you, he, she, etc.) in sentences, Spanish can omit them because the verb conjugation already indicates the subject. For instance: While in English you say "**I am a nurse**," in Spanish, you could perfectly omit the pronoun since the verb is conjugated for its particular form. So you could rather say "*Yo soy enfermera*" or simply "*Soy enfermera.*"
- **Question formation:** In English, questions are often formed by inverting the subject and the auxiliary verb (e.g., "*Is* he coming?"). In Spanish, questions are typically formed by adding an interrogative sign at the beginning and end of the sentence, with no inversion required, since the difference between a question and an affirmation is given by the signs in writing and by the tone spoken. For example: "Are you a nurse?" translates

to "*¿Eres enfermera?*" Without the interrogative signs and said with an affirmative tone, this same sentence becomes a statement: "*Eres enfermera*" (You are a nurse).

- **Double negatives**: While in English, double negatives are considered grammatically incorrect and cancel each other out (e.g., "I don't know nothing"). In Spanish, double negatives are standard and intensify the negation. For example: "*No sé nada*" has two negative words and literally translates to "I don't know nothing," but the real meaning is more like "I know nothing."

- **Adjective agreement:** As we just learned, in Spanish, adjectives must agree in gender and number with the nouns they modify. This means that if the noun is masculine and singular, the adjective must also be masculine and singular. In English, adjectives do not change based on the gender or number of the noun. For example: "The tall doctor" translates to "*El médico alto*" (masculine) or "*La médica alta*" (feminine). Likewise, "The tall doctors" would equally translate to "*Los doctores altos*" or "*Las doctoras altas.*"

VOCABULARY: THE BUILDING BLOCKS OF COMMUNICATION

Learning the basic Spanish vocabulary is the foundation for efficient communication with Spanish-speaking patients. Within the healthcare context, being able to convey fundamental phrases and terms not only demonstrates respect but also fosters a sense of trust and rapport. Here are essential Spanish phrases and words you should know, along with their English translations:

- *Hola*: Hello
- *¿Cómo está?*: How are you?
- *Gracias*: Thank you
- *Por favor*: Please
- *De acuerdo*: Okay
- *Lo siento*: I'm sorry
- *Necesito su ayuda*: I need your help
- *Está bien*: It's okay
- *¿Qué pasa?*: What's happening?
- *¿Puede explicar más?*: Can you explain more?
- *Aquí estoy para ayudar*: I'm here to help

Beyond greetings and courteous expressions, healthcare professionals should familiarize themselves with basic medical terms, as they are essential for patient assessment and care. In the following chapters, we will delve deeper into specific vocabulary for each medical area. Meanwhile, here are some crucial medical vocabulary words in Spanish and their English translations:

1. *Dolor*: Pain
2. *Fiebre*: Fever
3. *Respiración*: Breathing
4. *Sangre*: Blood
5. *Presión arterial*: Blood pressure
6. *Medicamento:* Medication
7. *Enfermedad*: Illness
8. *Lesión*: Injury
9. *Cirugía*: Surgery
10. *Radiografía*: X-ray
11. *Laboratorio*: Laboratory

12. *Emergencia*: Emergency

As a healthcare professional aiming to enhance your Spanish language skills for effective patient communication, you have a plethora of resources at your fingertips to practice and improve your abilities. Beyond formal lessons and structured courses, there are several avenues you can explore to integrate Spanish into your daily life and continuously elevate your language proficiency.

One engaging option is **Spanish-language news**. Tuning into Spanish news broadcasts or reading Spanish news articles allows you to stay updated on healthcare developments while refining your language skills. This exposure often includes interviews with medical experts, offering a firsthand encounter with medical terminology and its practical applications.

Consider seeking out **language exchange partners** who are native Spanish speakers. Offering your English language skills in exchange for conversational Spanish practice can be highly beneficial. Websites and platforms like *Tandem* and *ConversationExchange* facilitate these language exchange partnerships, creating opportunities for mutual learning and cultural exchange.

YouTube can be an unexpected but effective teacher. There are numerous **tutorials** available, covering various aspects of the Spanish language, including medical terminology and pronunciation. Visual aids can be particularly helpful in understanding complex concepts and mastering pronunciation.

For those looking to dive deeper into professional terminology, exploring **medical journals and publications** in Spanish can be instructive. Reading articles and publications related to healthcare in Spanish enables you to immerse yourself in specialized vocabulary and stay informed about medical advancements in Spanish-speaking regions.

Engaging with online **language communities** dedicated to learning Spanish is another fruitful avenue. Joining forums or communities provides a supportive environment where you can ask questions, share experiences, and practice conversational skills. Platforms like Reddit's r/Spanish and language-learning websites often have active communities eager to assist learners like you.

While *Duolingo* is a popular starting point, there are other **language-learning apps** to explore, such as *Babbel, Memrise*, or *Rosetta Stone*. These apps often offer more comprehensive courses that focus on speaking and listening skills, which are crucial for effective communication with patients.

Seeking out **language meetup groups** in your local area can provide opportunities for in-person interactions and cultural immersion. These groups often gather for social events or language practice sessions, fostering an environment where you can comfortably practice your conversational skills.

Lastly, keep an eye out for **Spanish-language films and TV shows** with subtitles. Watching them can be an enjoyable way to improve your listening skills while familiarizing yourself with colloquial language and cultural nuances.

Before delving into pronunciation and other topics, let me tell you that Spanish grammar is one of the most complex and extensive in the linguistic world. Here, for practical reasons, I have summarized the bases and foundations of the grammar of this language as much as possible so that you as a health professional can learn what is fundamental and necessary to begin communicating effectively with your patients as soon as possible. Even so, if you are interested in continuing to delve deeper into the grammatical foundations of Spanish, I recommend that you read my other book, *Learn Spanish for Adult Beginners: Speak Confidently & Impress Your Amigos - A No-Nonsense Guide to Quickly Learn Vocabulary, Common Phrases, and Master Pronunciation* (Mancilla, 2023), where you can learn more extensively everything related to this wonderful language, including its culture, nuances and diversity.

PRONUNCIATION: THE KEY TO BEING UNDERSTOOD

The correct pronunciation is paramount when communicating in a healthcare setting, as it not only facilitates effective interaction but also helps prevent misunderstandings that could potentially compromise patient care.

In Spanish, pronunciation generally follows a set of straightforward rules, making it accessible for English speakers. However, there are certain nuances to be aware of, especially for healthcare professionals aiming for clear and accurate communication.

One of the notable characteristics of Spanish pronunciation is that the letter "h"' is **always silent**. Unlike in English, where "h" can significantly impact word pronunciation, in Spanish, it is merely a placeholder. For instance, the word "hospital" in Spanish is pronounced "os-pee-tal," with no "h" sound.

Another letter that may pose a challenge for English speakers is "j," which sounds like the English "h." This can be particularly noticeable in words like "jalapeño," where the "j" is pronounced like "ha-lah-pee-nyo."

The Spanish "r" can be a bit tricky for English speakers as well. Unlike the English "r," which is pronounced with a rolling or flapping motion of the tongue, the Spanish "r" is a single flap of the tongue against the roof of the mouth. It's a stronger and quicker sound. To practice this sound, you can try repeating words like "*perro*" (dog) or "*carro*" (car).

Another letter you must be aware of is the "ñ". This one is a unique character in the Spanish language and represents a distinct sound. It is pronounced much like the "ny" in the English word "canyon." Whether discussing conditions like "*niños*" (children) or medical terms like "*niñera*" (babysitter), mastering the pronunciation of the "ñ" is crucial for healthcare professionals to convey information accurately and build rapport with Spanish-speaking patients—and avoid sounding funny.

Additionally, Spanish vowels are relatively simple, with **each vowel having only one sound**. This contrasts with English, where vowel sounds can vary significantly depending on the word. For example, in Spanish, "a" always sounds like the "a" in "father," "e" like the "e" in "red," "i" like the "ee" in "feet," "o" like the "o" in "go," and "u" like the "u" in "blue."

To practice and improve pronunciation, healthcare professionals can explore various resources beyond textbooks. Websites like Forvo offer a vast collection of words and phrases pronounced by native speakers. This can be a valuable tool to listen and mimic correct pronunciation. Additionally, Google Translate's audio function can provide a quick way to hear the correct pronunciation of words or phrases, making it a handy resource in daily practice.

Throughout this book you will frequently find the pronunciation of Spanish words given by the SPA Hispanic phonetics protocol. The idea is that you pronounce each syllable with the sound that you as an English speaker intuitively associate with that nomenclature. For example, the pronunciation of the word *"fiebre"* (fever) is given by: fee-eh-breh.

Let's expand on our current vocabulary implementing the correct pronunciation for each word:

- *Jeringa* (syringe): heh-reen-gah
- *Vendaje* (bandage): ben-dah-heh
- *Termómetro* (thermometer): tehr-moh-meh-troh
- *Tos* (cough): tohs
- *Mareo* (dizziness): mah-reh-oh
- *Vómito* (vomit): voh-mee-toh
- *Diarrea* (diarrhea): dee-ah-reh-ah
- *Picazón* (itching): pee-kah-sohn
- *Sarpullido* (rash): sahr-poo-yee-doh
- *Fatiga* (fatigue): fah-tee-gah
- *Estreñimiento* (constipation): es-treh-nyee-mee-ehn-toh
- *Sangrado* (bleeding): sahn-grah-doh

- *Inyección* (injection): een-yehk-see-ohn
- *Muletas* (crutches): moo-leh-tahs
- *Curita* (band-aid): koo-ree-tah

PRACTICE MAKES PERFECT

Let's talk about practice because, when it comes to learning a new language, it's all about practice and repetition. As a healthcare professional, you already understand the value of practice in your field, and the same principle applies here.

So, how can you practice your Spanish in a way that complements your busy schedule? Well, first and foremost, consider speaking simple Spanish phrases with your Spanish-speaking colleagues or patients (with their consent, of course). Just like any skill, practice makes perfect, and engaging in real conversations, even if they're brief, can boost your confidence and fluency.

But what if you're looking for more flexible options? Watching Spanish TV shows or listening to Spanish podcasts is an excellent choice. *Grey's Anatomy* is available in Spanish on Netflix. Why not give it a shot? It's a fun way to immerse yourself in the language while enjoying a familiar storyline. Additionally, there are fantastic podcasts like *Notes in Spanish* specifically designed for Spanish learners. These resources offer valuable insights into the language and culture, and you can listen to them during your commute or while exercising.

Remember, it's all about finding opportunities to integrate Spanish into your daily life. The more you practice, the more comfortable and confident you'll become in using Spanish in your healthcare interactions. So, seize those chances and you'll soon see your language skills improve!

A STEP TOWARDS CAREER ENHANCEMENT

Did you know that the demand for bilingual workers in the US has more than doubled between 2010 and 2015 (Colon, 2019)? That's a significant shift in the job market, and it's not slowing down. Being bilingual, especially in Spanish, can give you a competitive edge in your healthcare career. It opens doors to new opportunities, whether you're seeking a better position, aiming for a leadership role, or simply looking to stand out in a crowded field.

But there's more to it than just job prospects. Learning Spanish can lead to better job satisfaction as well. When you can communicate effectively with a wider range of patients, you're not just providing medical assistance; you're offering empathy, understanding, and a sense of trust. These qualities can profoundly impact patient outcomes and your own sense of fulfillment in your profession.

On a personal sphere, learning Spanish—like any other language —is a gateway to the richness of foreign cultures and art. Delving into the Spanish language allows you to connect with the soul of these cultures, appreciate the nuances of their traditions, and understand the profound beauty of their art, literature, and history. From the vibrant rhythms of salsa music to the marvelous tales written by Gabriel García Marquez and José Saramago, the Hispanic world is a treasure trove of creativity and passion.

As you immerse yourself in this language, you'll discover the joy of connecting with people from diverse backgrounds, exploring new cuisines, and experiencing the warmth of Hispanic hospitality, enriching a journey that broadens your horizons, ignites your curiosity, and fills your life with a deeper appreciation for the beauty of our global community.

So, as we conclude this chapter, I want to invite you to continue this journey with us. In the chapters ahead, we'll delve deeper into the intricacies of the Spanish language, cultural nuances, and practical strategies for improving your language skills. Whether you're just starting or already have a foundation in Spanish, this book is here to support you on your path to becoming a more confident and capable healthcare professional.

Te veo del otro lado.

EXERCISES AND PRACTICE

A. Complete the following sentences by selecting the correct subject pronoun in Spanish:

1. _____ *soy enfermera.*
2. _____ *necesito su ayuda.*
3. _____ *está en el hospital.*
4. _____ *tienes fiebre.*
5. _____ *estamos aquí para cuidarte.*

Translation:

1. I am a nurse.
2. I need your help.
3. He is in the hospital.
4. You have a fever.
5. We are here to take care of you.

Answers:

1. *Yo*
2. *Yo*
3. *Él*
4. *Tu*
5. *Nosotros/as*

B. Complete the following charts with the corresponding words and articles:

Article	Word in Spanish	English translation
El	hospital	The hospital
_____(1)	enfermera	The nurse (feminine)
Los	pacientes	_____(2) (masculine)
El	médico	The doctor (masculine)
La	medicina	The medicine
_____(3)	tratamiento	The treatment
Los	síntomas	The symptoms
Las	_____(4)	The X-rays
El	diagnóstico	The diagnosis
_____(5)	_____(6)	The prescription

Answers:

1. *La*
2. *The patients*
3. *El*
4. *Radiografías*
5. *La*
6. *Receta*

C. Translate the following sentences from English to Spanish, making sure to conjugate the verbs correctly according to the given tense and subject:

1. He helps the patient. (Present Simple):

   _____

2. They treated the injury. (Past Simple):

   _____

3. She explained the procedure. (Past Simple):

   _____

4. We are treating the illness. (Present Simple):

   _____

5. You will help the children. (Future Simple):

   _____

Answers:

1. *Él ayuda al paciente.*
2. *Ellos trataron la lesión.*
3. *Ella explicó el procedimiento.*
4. *Estamos tratando la enfermedad.*
5. *Tú ayudarás a los niños.*

D. Read the following medical terms and phrases in Spanish and repeat after the pronunciation guide to rehearse your pronunciation:

1. *Consulta médica* (kohn-sool-tah meh-dee-kah)
2. *Radiografía* (rah-dee-oh-grah-fee-ah)
3. *Enfermedad crónica* (ehn-fehr-meh-dahd kroh-nee-kah)

4. *Cirugía cardíaca* (see-roo-hee-ah kahr-dee-ah-kah)
5. *Tratamiento efectivo* (trah-tah-mee-ehn-toh eh-fehk-tee-boh)

Feel free to use online resources or language apps for correct pronunciation reference. These exercises will help you strengthen your foundational Spanish skills for healthcare communication. Enjoy practicing!

MEDICAL SPANISH DICTIONARY: A HEALTHCARE PROFESSIONAL'S GUIDE

N ow that you know the basics of Spanish grammar, you can begin to construct simple sentences. But before you can communicate with your patients and other Spanish speakers in the medical environment, you need to learn the terminology of the clinical field. We will dedicate the following pages to this.

This comprehensive guide offers not only translations of essential medical terms into Spanish but also provides pronunciation guides and examples of contextual usage. Whether you are a nurse, doctor, or any healthcare professional, this chapter aims to equip you with the linguistic tools necessary to communicate effectively with Spanish-speaking patients.

Vamos al lío.

GLOSSARY OF GENERAL HEALTH TERMS

General health terms serve as the foundation of any clear medical conversation. As healthcare professionals, you understand better than anyone the importance of precise and clear communication when discussing health-related matters with patients and their families. This section of our Medical Spanish Dictionary equips you with the fundamental vocabulary necessary for effective communication.

For instance, terms like "*salud*" (health), "*enfermedad*" (disease), and "*tratamiento*" (treatment) may seem basic. Still, they are the building blocks of understanding and conveying crucial information regarding a patient's well-being.

The knowledge of these terms allows you to grasp and convey information about a patient's health condition accurately. When a patient mentions "*salud*" or "*enfermedad*," you will immediately recognize that they are discussing their health or disease. For instance, if a patient says, "*Tengo una enfermedad del corazón*," you will readily understand that they have a heart disease.

However, it's not just about knowing these terms; correct pronunciation is equally necessary. For example, the word "*salud*" is pronounced as "sah-lood" in Spanish. Precise pronunciation is your key to preventing misunderstandings and ensuring that your patient interactions are as effective and compassionate as possible. So, let's delve into these essential terms, master their pronunciation, and empower you to navigate medical conversations with confidence and precision.

ANATOMY IN SPANISH: NAMING THE BODY PARTS

Let's start with the basics: the body parts. In the following table, you can find the most common limbs and body parts.

External body parts (*partes externas del cuerpo*):

Body part	Pronunciation	English translation
Cabeza	kah-beh-zah	Head
Cara	kah-rah	Face
Ojos	oh-hohs	Eyes
Oídos	oh-ee-dohs	Ears
Nariz	nah-reez	Nose
Boca	boh-kah	Mouth
Dientes	dee-ehn-tehs	Teeth
Cuello	kuh-eh-yoh	Neck
Hombros	ohm-brohs	Shoulders
Pecho	peh-choh	Chest
Espalda	ehs-pahl-dah	Back
Brazos	brah-zohs	Arms
Codos	coh-dohs	Elbows
Manos	mah-nohs	Hands
Dedos	dhe-dohs	Fingers
Vientre	bee-ehn-treh	Belly
Caderas	kah-deh-rahs	Hips
Piernas	pee-ehr-nahs	Legs

Rodillas	roh-dee-yahs	Knees
Pies	pee-ehs	Feet
Dedos de los pies	deh-dohs deh lohs pee-ehs	Toes

Mouth components (*componentes de la boca*):

Body part	Pronunciation	English translation
Labios	lah-bee-ohs	Lips
Dientes	dee-ehn-tehs	Teeth
Encías	ehn-see-ahs	Gums
Lengua	lehn-gwah	Tongue
Paladar	pah-lah-dahr	Palate
Amígdalas	ah-meeg-dah-lahs	Tonsils
Úvula	oo-buh-lah	Uvula
Saliva	sah-lee-vah	Saliva

Skeletal system (*sistema esquelético*):

Body part	Pronunciation	English translation
Huesos	weh-sohs	Bones
Cartílago	kar-tee-lah-go	Cartilage
Articulaciones	ahr-tee-koo-lah-syo-nes	Joints
Tejido nervioso	teh-hee-doh ner-vee-oh-so	Nervous tissue
Craneo	krah-neh-oh	Skull
Columna vertebral	koh-loo-mnah vehr-teh-brahl	Spine
Costillas	kohs-tee-yahs	Ribs
Esternón	ehs-tehr-nohn	Sternum

Cardiovascular system (*sistema cardiovascular*):

Body part	Pronunciation	English translation
Corazón	koh-rah-zohn	Heart
Vasos Sanguíneos	bah-sohs sahn-ghee-neh-ohs	Blood Vessels
Arterias	ahr-teh-ree-ahs	Arteries
Venas	veh-nahs	Veins

Respiratory system (*sistema respiratorio*):

Body part	Pronunciation	English translation
Pulmones	pool-moh-nes	Lungs
Tráquea	trah-keh-ah	Trachea
Bronquios	brohn-kee-ohs	Bronchi
Diafragma	dee-ah-frag-mah	Diaphragm

Nervous system (*sistema nervioso*):

Body part	Pronunciation	English translation
Cerebro	seh-reh-broh	Brain
Médula Espinal	meh-doo-lah ehs-pee-nahl	Spinal Cord
Nervios	nehr-bee-ohs	Nerves
Músculos	moo-skoo-lohs	Muscles

Digestive system (*sistema digestivo*):

Body part	Pronunciation	English translation
Estómago	ehs-toh-mah-goh	Stomach
Intestino Delgado	een-tehs-tee-noh dehl-gah-doh	Small Intestine
Intestino Grueso	een-tehs-tee-noh grew-eh-soh	Large Intestine
Hígado	ee-gah-doh	Liver
Vesícula Biliar	veh-see-koo-lah bee-lee-ahr	Gallbladder
Páncreas	pahn-kreh-ahs	Pancreas

Urinary system (*sistema urinario*):

Body part	Pronunciation	English translation
Riñones	ree-nyee-oh-nehs	Kidneys
Vejiga	veh-hee-gah	Bladder
Uretra	oo-reh-trah	Urethra

Body secretions and fluids (*secreciones y fluidos del cuerpo*):

Secretion/Fluid	Pronunciation	English translation
Sangre	sahn-greh	Blood
Saliva	sah-lee-vah	Saliva
Lágrimas	lah-gree-mahs	Tears
Sudor	soo-dohr	Sweat
Orina	oh-ree-nah	Urine
Mucosidad	moo-koh-see-dahd	Mucus
Pus	poos	Pus
Ácido Gástrico	ah-see-doh gah-stree-koh	Gastric Acid

Practice this vocabulary and if it helps you, I recommend that you look for images of the body and label them. This will be of enormous help to you since having graphic support increases your chances of learning and correctly associating words with their meaning. You can choose different label colors for the different systems and parts of the body, making the association clearer and easier for your brain to internalize (Dzulkifli & Mustafar, 2013).

Before continuing, let's put this new vocabulary to use by applying it to the following example:

- *Paciente: ¡Hola, doctor! Me **siento mal**. Tengo **dolor** en todo el cuerpo y me siento muy **cansado**.*

(Hello, doctor! I'm not feeling well. I have pain all over my body and I feel very tired)

- **Doctor:** *Hola, ¿desde cuándo siente estos **síntomas**? ¿Puede describir dónde siente el dolor?*

(Hello, since when have you been experiencing these symptoms? Can you describe where you feel the pain?)

- **P:** *He tenido estos síntomas durante una semana. El dolor está en mis **articulaciones** y **músculos**, especialmente en las **piernas** y los **brazos**.*

(I've had these symptoms for a week. The pain is in my joints and muscles, especially in my legs and arms.)

- **D:** *Entiendo. Vamos a hacer algunas **pruebas**. ¿Ha tenido **fiebre** o **dolor de garganta**?*

(I understand. We'll run some tests. Have you had a fever or a sore throat?)

- **P:** *Sí, he tenido fiebre y dolor de garganta también.*

(Yes, I've had a fever and a sore throat as well.)

- **D:** *Gracias por la información. Vamos a hacer un **análisis de sangre** para entender mejor lo que está ocurriendo. También revisaremos su garganta y articulaciones en detalle.*

(Thank you for the information. We'll do some blood tests to better understand what's happening. We'll also examine your throat and joints in detail.)

DECODING MEDICAL PROCEDURES IN SPANISH

The next thing we will address will be the different medical procedures that we can perform on the patient. For reasons of practicality and so that you can consult it when you need it, I have arranged them in alphabetical order and added their translation and correct pronunciation.

Procedure	Spanish translation	Spanish pronunciation
Biopsy	Biopsia	Bee-ohp-see-ah
Blood Test	Análisis de Sangre	Ah-nah-lee-sees deh Sahn-greh
Chemotherapy	Quimioterapia	Kee-mee-oh-teh-rah-pee-ah
Colonoscopy	Colonoscopia	Koh-loh-nohs-koh-pee-ah
Dental Procedure	Procedimiento Dental	Pro-seh-dee-mee-ehn-toh Dehn-tahl
Dialysis	Diálisis	Dee-ah-lee-sees
Endoscopy	Endoscopia	Ehn-dohs-koh-pee-ah
Examination	Examen	Eh-kzah-mehn
Heart Transplant	Trasplante de Corazón	Trahs-plahn-teh deh Koh-rah-sohn
MRI	Resonancia Magnética	Reh-soh-nahn-see-ah mahg-neh-tee-kah
Physical Therapy	Terapia Física	Teh-rah-pee-ah Fee-see-kah
Radiation Therapy	Radioterapia	Rah-dee-oh-teh-rah-pee-ah
Surgery	Cirugía	See-roo-hee-ah
Vaccination	Vacunación	Bah-koo-nah-see-ohn
X-ray	Radiografía	Rah-dee-oh-grah-fee-ah

From the following conversation between a nurse and a mother, you can begin to generate an intuition of how to use these words:

- **Enfermera:** *Hola, soy la enfermera Laura. ¿Usted es la madre de Juan?*

(Hello, I'm Nurse Laura. Are you Juan's mother?)

- **Madre:** *Sí, soy su madre. ¿Cómo está mi hijo?*

(Yes, I'm his mother. How is my son?)

- **E:** *Su hijo está estable en este momento, pero tuvo un **accidente** en bicicleta. Tiene algunas **lesiones** en el cuerpo y una **cadera rota**. Necesitamos hacer una **radiografía**, una **transfusión de sangre** y una **resonancia magnética** en su cabeza antes de la **cirugía** para reparar su hueso.*

(Your son is stable at the moment, but he had a bike accident. He has some injuries on his body and a broken hip. We need to do an X-ray, a blood transfusion, and an MRI on his head before the surgery to repair his bone.)

- **M:** *¡Dios mío, eso suena grave! ¿Está sufriendo mucho **dolor**?*

(Oh my God, that sounds serious! Is he in a lot of pain?)

- **E:** *Estamos controlando su dolor y lo mantendremos cómodo. Estamos haciendo todo lo posible por su **bienestar**.*

(We are managing his pain and we will keep him comfortable. We are doing everything we can for his well-being.)

- **M:** *Gracias por cuidar de mi hijo. ¿Puedo verlo antes de los* **procedimientos?**

(Thank you for taking care of my son. Can I see him before the procedures?)

- **E:** *Claro, le permitiremos verlo antes de que comencemos con los procedimientos médicos. Estamos aquí para apoyarlos en todo momento.*

(Of course, we will allow you to see him before we start with the medical procedures. We are here to support you both at all times.)

PHARMACOLOGICAL VOCABULARY: SPANISH FOR MEDICATIONS

This section will introduce you to the pharmacological vocabulary you need to give prescriptions and medications effectively to your patients.

While you may not be expected to become a full-fledged pharmacist, having a grasp of medication-related terms will significantly enhance your ability to communicate treatment plans to Spanish-speaking patients. So, let's move on to ensuring that no language barrier stands in the way of delivering the best care possible.

Let's start by addressing some of the most common terms related to medications and prescriptions.

Spanish term	Pronunciation	English translation
Analgésico	ah-nahl-geh-see-koh	Analgesic (painkiller)
Antibiótico	ahn-tee-bee-oh-tee-koh	Antibiotic
Anticoagulante	ahn-tee-koh-ah-goo-lahn-teh	Anticoagulant
Contraindicaciones	kohn-trah-yn-dee-kah-syoh-nehs	Contraindications
Dosificación	doh-see-fee-kah-see-ohn	Dosage
Dosis	doh-sees	Dose
Efectos secundarios	eh-fehk-tohs seh-koon-dah-ree-ohs	Side effects
Farmacia	fahr-mah-see-ah	Pharmacy
Genérico	heh-neh-ree-koh	Generic
Ingredientes	een-greh-dee-ehn-tes	Ingredients
Insulina	een-soo-lee-nah	Insulin
Interacciones	een-ter-ahk-syoh-nehss	Interactions
Medicina	meh-dee-see-nah	Medicine
Pastilla	pahs-tee-yah	Pill
Posología	poh-soh-loh-hee-ah	Dosage instructions
Receta	reh-seh-tah	Prescription
Receta médica	reh-seh-tah meh-dee-kah	Medical prescription
Suspensión	soo-spehn-syohn	Suspension
Jarabe	hah-rah-beh	Syrup

Now let's look at some examples applying those terms:

- *Necesita tomar este **analgésico** para el dolor* (You need to take this painkiller for the pain.)
- *¿Es este un **antibiótico** para mi infección?* (Is this an antibiotic for my infection?)
- *La **insulina** es importante para controlar la diabetes.* (Insulin is important for controlling diabetes.)
- *¿Puedo recoger mi **medicina** en la **farmacia**?* (Can I pick up my medicine at the pharmacy?)
- *Esta es una **receta** para su medicina* (This is a prescription for your medicine.)

EXERCISES AND PRACTICE

A. Read and complete the translation below:

Paciente: Hola, doctor. Me siento mal. Tengo dolor de cabeza y fiebre desde ayer. Además, mis músculos y articulaciones me duelen mucho.

Doctor: Entiendo, siento que te sientas mal. Vamos a ver qué está pasando. ¿Puedes decirme más sobre tu dolor de cabeza? ¿Es un dolor punzante o constante?

P: Es constante, como una presión en la frente. También me duele la garganta y tengo tos.

D: Gracias por la información. Parece que tienes varios síntomas. Vamos a revisarte. Primero, midamos tu temperatura. Luego, haremos algunos exámenes para determinar la causa de tus síntomas.

P: ¿Necesitaré tomar medicamentos?

D: Eso dependerá de lo que encontremos en los exámenes. Lo importante ahora es obtener un diagnóstico preciso. Trabajaré contigo para ayudarte a sentirte mejor. Por favor, espera un momento mientras preparo los exámenes.

Translation

P: Hello, doctor. I don't feel well. I have a _____ (1) and fever since yesterday. Also, my muscles and _____ (2) hurt a lot.

D: I understand, I'm sorry you are feeling bad. Let's see what's happening. Can you tell me more about your headache? Is it a stabbing or constant pain?

P: It's constant, like pressure on the forehead. My _____ (3) also hurts and I have a cough.

D: Thanks for the information. It sounds like you have several symptoms. Let's check you out. First, let's measure your temperature. Then, we will do some _____ (4) to determine the cause of your symptoms.

P: Will I need to take _____ (5)?

D: That will depend on what we find in the exams. The important thing now is to obtain an accurate _____ (6). I will work with you to help you feel better. Please wait a moment while I prepare for the exams.

Answers:

1. headache
2. joints

3. throat
4. tests
5. medication
6. diagnosis

B. Develop a set of flashcards with medical terms in Spanish on one side and their English translations on the other. Use these flashcards for self-testing and review.

DIALOGUES FOR DIAGNOSIS: SPANISH FOR PATIENT INTERACTION

As we have realized through this exploration, for healthcare professionals, the ability to communicate with patients is crucial in providing the best care possible. However, when language barriers come into play, these interactions can become challenging. This chapter aims to bridge that gap by offering practical Spanish phrases and dialogues specifically tailored for various medical scenarios, empowering healthcare professionals to provide more effective and empathetic care for Spanish-speaking patients.

A nurse friend once regaled me with a story from her own experience. In a situation where a patient required immediate attention for what seemed to be a severe symptom, an interpreter was called to facilitate communication. However, a misunderstanding arose between the patient, the interpreter, and the medical staff regarding the symptom's nature and severity. This incident highlighted the critical need for healthcare professionals to have autonomy in communicating with their patients, without solely relying on interpreters. To avoid those scenarios, I aim to equip you with the skills and confidence to navigate such scenarios smoothly, ensuring that both you and your patients understand each other clearly.

BREAKING THE ICE: INITIAL PATIENT INTERACTION

Initiating a medical conversation with a Spanish-speaking patient is the first step in establishing a rapport and ensuring a positive healthcare experience. This initial contact sets the tone for the entire interaction, making it essential to begin on a strong note.

To create a warm and welcoming atmosphere, start with simple greetings such as "*Buenos días*" (good morning) or "*Hola, ¿cómo puedo ayudarle hoy?*" (Hello, how can I help you today?). These greetings convey respect and set the stage for a productive conversation.

Asking about the patient's overall feeling or well-being is a crucial part of the initial interaction. Use phrases like "*¿Cómo se siente hoy?*" (How are you feeling today?) to assess their current state. Additionally, inquiring about pain levels with "*En una escala del 1 al 10, cuanto dolor siente hoy?*" (On a scale of 1 to 10, how much pain are you feeling today?) is essential to understanding their discomfort accurately.

Encourage open dialogue by posing open-ended questions. For example, "*¿Puede contarme más sobre...?*" (Can you tell me more about...?) invites patients to share additional details about their symptoms or concerns. This approach fosters a sense of collaboration, where patients actively participate in their healthcare.

Also, it's crucial to use words of reassurance to convey empathy and understanding. Phrases like "*Entiendo lo que está pasando*" (I understand what you're going through) can help patients feel seen and heard, reducing anxiety and building trust. Expressing affirmations like "*Estamos aquí para ayudarle*" (We are here to help you) reassures patients that they are in capable and compassionate hands, fostering a positive patient-provider relationship from the outset.

Here you have a practical chart, useful to have on hand, with some useful expressions to break the ice and establish accurate and empathetic contact with the patient:

Spanish expression	Pronunciation	English translation
Buenos días	Bweh-nohs dee-ahs	Good morning
Hola, ¿cómo puedo ayudarle hoy?	Oh-lah, koh-moh pweh-doh ah-yoo-dahr-leh oh-ee	Hello, how can I help you today?
¿Cómo se siente hoy?	Koh-moh seh syehn-teh oh-ee	How are you feeling today?
En una escala del 1 al 10, cuanto dolor siente hoy?	Ehn oo-nah ehs-kah-lah dehl ooh-noh ahl dee-ehz, kwahn-toh doh-lohr syehn-teh oh-ee	On a scale of 1 to 10, how much pain are you feeling today?
¿Puede contarme más sobre...?	Poo-eh-deh kohn-tahr-meh mahs soh-breh...?	Can you tell me more about...?
Entiendo lo que está pasando	Ehn-tee-ehn-doh loh keh eh-stah pah-sahn-doh	I understand what you're going through
Estamos aquí para ayudarle	Ehs-tah-mohs ah-kee pah-rah ah-yoo-dahr-leh	We are here to help you

SPEAKING OF SYMPTOMS: DISCUSSING MEDICAL
HISTORY AND CURRENT SYMPTOMS

As you know, understanding a patient's medical history and
current symptoms is essential for an accurate diagnosis and
effective treatment. When communicating with Spanish-
speaking patients, it's crucial to ask the right questions and
actively listen to their responses.

To start the discussion about a patient's medical history, it's
essential to use polite and open-ended questions to gather relevant information. Here are some phrases to use:

- *¿Puede contarme sobre su historial médico?* (Can you tell me
  about your medical history?)
- *¿Ha tenido problemas médicos en el pasado?* (Have you had
  medical problems in the past?)
- *¿Alguna vez ha sido hospitalizado?* (Have you ever been
  hospitalized?)

When discussing the patient's current symptoms, it's important
to ask specific and direct questions to pinpoint their condition
accurately. Here are some helpful phrases for this part of the
conversation:

- *¿Cuándo empezaron los síntomas?* (When did the symptoms
  start?)
- *¿Dónde siente dolor?* (Where do you feel pain?)
- *¿Cómo describiría la intensidad del dolor?* (How would you
  describe the intensity of the pain?)

Active listening is a vital skill when discussing medical history and symptoms with patients. After the patient provides their responses, it's essential to confirm your understanding to ensure clarity and accuracy. Use phrases like:

- *Si entiendo correctamente, usted está experimentando...* (If I understand correctly, you are experiencing...)
- *Entendido. Entonces, haremos lo siguiente...* (Understood. So, we'll do the following...)

To complete the patient's medical profile, it's important to ask about any medications they are currently taking. Here are relevant phrases:

- *¿Está tomando algún medicamento actualmente?* (Are you currently taking any medication?)
- *¿Cuántas veces al día toma este medicamento?* (How many times a day do you take this medication?)

Let's continue building the wall of knowledge of this wonderful language. In previous sections, we armed ourselves with the learning of basic words to understand which part of the patient's body is affected and what treatments we can conduct on them. Now, we will examine what potential symptoms the patient may show. Below are the most common symptoms:

Spanish symptom	Pronunciation	English translation
Dolor abdominal	doh-lohr ahb-doh-mee-nahl	Abdominal pain
Hemorragia/sangrado	eh-moh-rah-hee-ah/sahn-grah-doh	Bleeding
Dolor en el pecho	doh-lohr ehn ehl peh-choh	Chest pain
Escalofríos	ehs-kah-loh-free-ohs	Chills
Estreñimiento	eh-streh-nyee-mee-ehn-toh	Constipation
Dificultad para respirar	dee-fee-kool-tahd pah-rah rehs-pee-rahr	Difficulty breathing
Mareos	mah-reh-ohs	Dizziness
Sudoración excesiva	soo-doh-rah-see-ohn ehk-seh-see-vah	Excessive sweating
Sangrado de encías	sahn-grah-doh deh ehn-see-ahs	Gum bleeding
Ronquera	ron-keh-rah	Hoarseness
Inflamación	een-flah-mah-see-on	Swelling
Irritación	ee-ree-tah-see-ohn	Irritation
Secreción nasal	seh-kreh-see-ohn nah-sahl	Nasal discharge
Picazón en la piel	pee-kah-sohn ehn lah pee-ehl	Skin itching
Vértigo	vehr-tee-goh	Vertigo

Here's a chart with common **types of pain** in Spanish, their pronunciation, and English translations:

Spanish term	Pronunciation	English translation
Agudo	ah-goo-doh	Acute/sharp
Crónico	kroh-nee-koh	Chronic
Punzante	poon-sahn-teh	Piercing, stabbing
Intenso	een-ten-soh	Intense
Leve	leh-veh	Mild
Persistente	pehr-sis-ten-teh	Persistent
Intermitente	een-ter-mee-ten-teh	Intermittent
Opresivo	oh-preh-see-voh	Oppressive, crushing
Agobiante	ah-goh-bee-ahn-teh	Overwhelming
Lancinante	lahn-see-nahn-teh	Lancinating
Ardiente	ahr-dee-ehn-teh	Burning
Molesto	moh-lehs-toh	Annoying
Penetrante	peh-neh-trahn-teh	Penetrating
Incómodo	een-koh-moh-doh	Uncomfortable

Below, you can check some examples of potential real scenarios where patients describe their current symptoms:

- **Patient:** *Buenos días, doctor. Desde ayer he estado sintiendo un dolor agudo en el pecho y dificultad para respirar. También tengo sudores fríos. No sé qué está pasando.*

Translation: Good morning, doctor. Since yesterday, I've been feeling sharp chest pain and difficulty breathing. I also have cold sweats. I don't know what's happening.

- *Patient: Hola, enfermera. Tengo fiebre alta desde hace tres días, me duele la garganta y tengo congestión nasal. Además, tengo dolor en todo el cuerpo.*

Translation: Hi, nurse. I've had a high fever for three days, my throat hurts, and I have a stuffy nose. Also, my whole body aches.

- *Patient: Doctor, desde la semana pasada he notado que tengo sangre en las heces y me siento cansado todo el tiempo. Además, he perdido peso sin razón aparente.*

Translation: Doctor, since last week, I've noticed blood in my stool and I feel tired all the time. Also, I've lost weight for no apparent reason.

- *Patient: Buenas tardes. Me desmayé en el trabajo hoy, y me duele mucho la cabeza desde hace varios días. Además, tengo visión borrosa y mareos frecuentes.*

Translation: Good afternoon. I fainted at work today and I've had a severe headache for several days. Also, I have blurry vision and frequent dizziness.

- *Patient: Enfermera, estoy experimentando un fuerte dolor abdominal en el lado derecho, y siento náuseas constantes. También tengo fiebre y escalofríos.*

Translation: Nurse, I'm experiencing severe abdominal pain on the right side and I have constant nausea. I also have a fever and chills.

READING THE RESULTS: EXPLAINING DIAGNOSES AND TREATMENT PLANS

Clear communication is crucial when explaining diagnoses and treatment plans to patients, especially when language barriers may exist. Effective communication ensures that patients fully understand their medical condition and the proposed course of treatment. Healthcare professionals can use specific phrases and techniques to facilitate this process.

When discussing diagnoses, it's essential to be direct and clear. Start by using phrases like *"Los resultados muestran que usted tiene..."* (The results show that you have…). This provides patients with a straightforward introduction to their diagnosis, avoiding any ambiguity.

Explaining treatment plans should also involve simple, easy-to-understand language. Use phrases such as *"El plan de tratamiento incluirá..."* (The treatment plan will include…) or *"Es importante que usted..."* (It is important that you…) to outline the proposed course of action. Avoid medical jargon and technical terms unless the patient is familiar with them.

Always check for understanding and encourage questions from the patient. After explaining the diagnosis and treatment plan, ask, *"¿Entiende lo que acabo de explicar?"* (Do you understand what I just explained?). This step is crucial to ensure that the patient comprehends the information provided. If there is any uncertainty or confusion, it can be addressed promptly.

Furthermore, it's essential to actively encourage patients to ask questions or express any concerns they may have. Use phrases like "*¿Tiene alguna pregunta o preocupación?*" (Do you have any questions or concerns?). This not only invites patients to seek clarification but also demonstrates your commitment to their well-being and comfort.

Here's a chart with key expressions for explaining diagnoses and treatment plans to patients in Spanish, along with their pronunciation and English translations:

Spanish expression	Pronunciation	English translation
Los resultados muestran que usted tiene...	lohs reh-sool-tah-dohs moo-ehs-trahn keh oos-tehd tyeh-neh...	The results show that you have...
El plan de tratamiento incluirá...	ehl plahn deh trah-tah-mee-ehn-toh een-kloo-ee-rah...	The treatment plan will include...
Es importante que usted...	ehs eem-pohr-tahn-teh keh oos-tehd...	It is important that you...
¿Entiende lo que acabo de explicar?	ehn-tee-ehn-deh loh keh ah-kah-boh deh ehks-plee-kahr...	Do you understand what I just explained?
¿Tiene alguna pregunta o preocupación?	tee-eh-neh al-goo-nah preh-goon-tah o preh-oh-koo-pah-see-ohn	Do you have any questions or concerns?

Le explicaré su diagnóstico más detalladamente.	leh ehks-plee-kah-reh soo dyahg-nohs-tee-koh mahs deh-tah-yah-dah-mehn-teh	I will explain your diagnosis in more detail.
El tratamiento tiene como objetivo...	el trah-tah-mee-ehn-toh tee-eh-neh koh-moh oh-bheh-tee-voh	The treatment aims to...
Para su bienestar, es fundamental seguir el tratamiento.	pah-rah soo bee-ehn-ehs-tahr, ehs foon-dah-mehn-tahl seh-gheer el trah-tah-mee-ehn-toh	For your well-being, it is essential to follow the treatment.
¿Hay algo que no comprende o le preocupa?	ay ahl-goh keh noh kohm-prehn-deh o leh preh-oh-koo-pah	Is there anything you don't understand or are concerned about?

In the following chart, you can find some of the most common diagnoses ordered alphabetically. This chart can be really handy when explaining your patients their clinical situation:

Diagnosis	Spanish translation	Spanish pronunciation
Allergy	Alergia	ah-lehr-hee-ah
Arthritis	Artritis	ahr-tree-tees
Asthma	Asma	ahs-mah
Bronchitis	Bronquitis	brohn-kee-teess
Cancer	Cáncer	kahn-sehr
Diabetes	Diabetes	dee-ah-beh-tehs
Epilepsy	Epilepsia	eh-pee-lep-see-ah
Fracture	Fractura	frahk-too-rah
Gastritis	Gastritis	gahs-tree-tees
Hypertension	Hipertensión	ee-pehr-tehn-see-ohn
Infection	Infección	een-fehk-see-ohn
Migraine	Migraña	mee-grah-nyah
Pneumonia	Neumonía	neh-oo-moh-nee-ah
Pregnancy	Embarazo	ehm-bah-rah-so
Rheumatism	Reumatismo	reh-oo-mah-tees-moh
Stroke	Accidente cerebrovascular (ACV)	ahk-see-den-teh seh-reh-broh-vahs-koo-lahr (ah seh beh)
Ulcer	Úlcera	ool-seh-rah
Anemia	Anemia	ah-neh-mee-ah
Hypothyroidism	Hipotiroidismo	ee-poh-tee-roy-dees-moh
Osteoporosis	Osteoporosis	ohs-teh-oh-poh-roh-sees

In the following chart, you'll find treatments and medical procedures along with their proper pronunciation and translation:

Treatment/Procedure	Spanish translation	Spanish pronunciation
Chemotherapy	Quimioterapia	kee-mee-oh-teh-rah-pee-ah
Dental extraction	Extracción dental	ehks-trahk-syon dehn-tahl
Dialysis	Diálisis	dee-ah-lee-sees
Electrocardiogram (ECG or EKG)	Electrocardiograma	eh-lehk-troh-kahr-dee-oh-grah-mah
Endoscopy	Endoscopia	ehn-dohs-koh-pee-ah
Hernia repair	Reparación de hernia	reh-pah-rah-see-ohn deh ehr-nyah
Joint replacement	Reemplazo de articulación	reh-ehm-plah-soh deh ahr-tee-koo-lah-syon
Laser surgery	Cirugía láser	see-roo-hee-ah lah-sehr
Mammogram	Mamografía	mah-moh-grah-fee-ah
Organ transplant	Trasplante de órganos	trahs-plan-teh deh ohr-gah-nohs
Physical examination	Examen físico	ehk-sah-mehn fee-see-koh
Physical therapy	Terapia física	teh-rah-pee-ah fee-see-kah
Respiratory therapy	Terapia respiratoria	teh-rah-pee-ah reh-spee-rah-toh-ree-ah
Vaccination	Vacunación	vah-koo-nah-see-ohn

Keep in mind that in the previous chapter, we already addressed some of the most common treatments and medical procedures, so you can check those charts to complete the vocabulary.

The following dialogs will provide you with examples of use for these new words:

Scenario 1:

Doctor: Buenas tardes, señor García. Los resultados muestran que usted tiene diabetes tipo 2. (Good afternoon, Mr. García. The results show that you have type 2 diabetes.)

Paciente: ¿Diabetes? ¿Qué significa eso? (Diabetes? What does that mean?)

D: Significa que su cuerpo tiene dificultades para controlar el azúcar en la sangre. Pero no se preocupe, podemos tratarla. (It means that your body has trouble controlling blood sugar. But don't worry, we can treat it.)

Scenario 2:

Enfermero: Hola, señora López. Quiero informarle que después de las pruebas, hemos confirmado que tiene hipertensión. (Hello, Mrs. López. I want to inform you that after the tests, we have confirmed that you have hypertension.)

Paciente: Entendido, ¿qué debo hacer ahora? (Understood, what should I do now?)

E: Necesitará cambios en su dieta y medicamentos para controlarla. Estamos aquí para ayudarle en cada paso del camino. (You'll need changes in your diet and medications to control it. We are here to help you every step of the way.)

Scenario 3:

Doctor: Buen día, señor Rodríguez. Los análisis muestran que tiene una infección en el tracto urinario. (Good morning, Mr. Rodríguez. The tests show that you have a urinary tract infection.)

Le recetaré antibióticos para tratarla, y es importante que tome todos los medicamentos según las indicaciones. (I will prescribe antibiotics to treat it, and it's important that you take all the medications as directed.)

Scenario 4:

Enfermera: Señorita Pérez. Los exámenes de sangre revelan que tiene anemia. (Miss Pérez. Blood tests reveal that you have anemia.)

Paciente: Anemia, ¿qué implica eso? (Anemia, what does that entail?)

E: Significa que sus glóbulos rojos están bajos, lo que puede causar fatiga. Le daremos suplementos de hierro y pautas dietéticas para mejorar su salud. (It means that your red blood cell count is low, which can lead to fatigue. We will provide iron supplements and dietary guidelines to improve your health.)

UNDER PRESSURE: HANDLING EMERGENCIES AND CRITICAL SITUATIONS

Imagine a scenario in which a patient suddenly experiences severe chest pain. You, as a healthcare professional, spring into action. In such situations, there's no time for lengthy explanations. Instead, you need to use short, clear instructions. Phrases like *"Necesito que se calme y respire profundamente"* (I need you to calm down and breathe deeply) can help the patient focus and alleviate their anxiety. By communicating the urgency of the situation, you prepare the patient for the actions you're about to take. For instance, "*Vamos a llevarle a la sala de urgencias ahora*" (We are going to take you to the emergency room now) conveys a sense of immediacy and the need for swift action.

As your experiences have shown you, emergencies can be frightening for patients and their families. Providing reassurance is a crucial aspect of communication. In the midst of chaos, conveying empathy and care can make all the difference. Phrases like "*Estamos haciendo todo lo posible para ayudarle*" (We are doing everything we can to help you) reassure the patient that they are in capable hands. It helps them understand that their well-being is the top priority.

During emergencies, it's not just the patient who needs information; their family often seeks updates as well. Effective communication means keeping both the patient and their loved ones informed. For example, when the doctor is on the way, you can say, "*El médico estará aquí pronto*" (The doctor will be here soon). This lets the patient and their family know that help is on the way and provides them with a sense of relief.

Furthermore, when medical tests and procedures are being conducted, patients and their families may be anxious and uncertain about the situation. By saying, "*Estamos haciendo pruebas para entender mejor lo que está pasando*" (We are doing tests to better understand what is going on), you offer transparency and a glimpse into the medical process. It empowers the patient and their family with knowledge, reducing anxiety and enhancing trust in the healthcare team.

In critical situations, every word you say matters. It can comfort, reassure, and provide clarity. Effective communication is not just about relaying information; it's about maintaining trust and compassion, even in the most challenging of circumstances.

Here's a chart including the expressions for handling emergencies and critical situations in Spanish, along with their English translations and pronunciations:

Spanish phrase	English translation	Spanish pronunciation
Necesito que se calme y respire profundamente	I need you to calm down and breathe deeply	neh-seh-see-toh keh seh kahl-meh ee rehs-pee-reh proh-foon-dah-mehn-teh
Vamos a llevarle a la sala de urgencias ahora	We are going to take you to the emergency room now	vah-mohs ah yeh-vahr-leh ah lah sah-lah deh oor-hehn-see-ahs ah-oh-rah
Estamos haciendo todo lo posible para ayudarle	We are doing everything we can to help you	ehs-tah-mohs ah-see-ehn-doh toh-doh loh poh-see-bleh pah-rah ah-yoo-dahr-leh
El médico estará aquí pronto	The doctor will be here soon	ehl meh-dee-koh ehs-tah-rah ah-kee prohn-toh
Estamos haciendo pruebas para entender mejor lo que está pasando	We are doing tests to better understand what is going on	ehs-tah-mohs ah-see-ehn-doh prweh-bahs pah-rah ehn-tehn-dehr meh-hor loh keh ehs-tah pah-sahn-doh

EXERCISES AND PRACTICE

A. Read the following dialogue and then complete the translation in Spanish with the missing words:

Healthcare Professional (HP): Good morning. How can I assist you today?

Patient (P): Good morning. I'm here because I don't feel very well.

HP: I understand. What are your symptoms?

P: I have a headache, a fever, and chest pain.

HP: I'm sorry to hear that. Let's figure out what's going on. When did these symptoms start?

P: They began yesterday afternoon. I got worried because the chest pain is new for me.

HP: Thank you for sharing that. Have you had similar health issues in the past?

P: No, I've never had this before. I'm a little scared.

HP: I understand why you would be concerned. We're here to help you. We're going to run some tests to better understand what's happening. Is there anything else you'd like to tell me about your symptoms?

P: No, that's all for now.

HP: Very well. We'll take care of you and determine the cause of your symptoms. If you have any questions or concerns at any time, please don't hesitate to let us know.

Translation:

HP: Buenos días. ¿Cómo puedo ayudarle hoy?

P: Buenos días. Estoy aquí porque no me siento muy bien.

HP: Entiendo. ¿Cuáles son sus _____ (1)?

P: Me _____(2) y tengo _____(3). Además, tengo dolor en el _____(4).

HP: Siento escuchar eso. Vamos a averiguar lo que está pasando. ¿Desde cuándo empezaron estos síntomas?

P: Empezaron ayer por la tarde. Me preocupé porque el dolor en el pecho es nuevo para mí.

HP: Gracias por compartir eso. ¿Ha tenido _____ (5) similares en el pasado?

P: No, nunca había tenido esto antes. Estoy un poco asustado.

HP: Entiendo por qué estaría preocupado. _____ (6). Vamos a hacer algunas _____ (7) para comprender mejor lo que está sucediendo. ¿Alguna otra cosa que quiera contarme sobre sus síntomas?

P: No, eso es todo por ahora.

HP: Muy bien. Vamos a cuidar de usted y averiguar la causa de sus síntomas. Si tiene alguna pregunta o preocupación en cualquier momento, no dude en decírnoslo.

Answers:

1. *síntomas*
2. *duele la cabeza*
3. *fiebre*
4. *pecho*
5. *problemas de salud*
6. *Estamos aquí para ayudarle*
7. *pruebas*

B. Read the following dialogue between a doctor and a worried family about the situation of a loved one. Try to read out loud and, if possible, ask a native speaker to record it for you so you get familiar with the pronunciation and accent. The English translation is available below, and you can check it to reinforce the learned vocabulary:

HP: Buenos días, familia. Soy la doctora Green, y estamos atendiendo a su ser querido en este momento. Entiendo que están preocupados, pero permítanme brindarles información importante.

Family: ¿Cómo está? ¿Qué está pasando?

HP: Entendemos que esto es angustiante. Su familiar está siendo atendida por nuestro equipo médico. Estamos realizando pruebas para determinar la causa de su malestar. Por favor, siéntanse tranquilos sabiendo que estamos haciendo todo lo posible para ayudarle.

F: ¿Puede decirnos qué está sucediendo?

HP: Claro. Su ser querido ha experimentado un dolor en el pecho y dificultad para respirar. Estos síntomas son preocupantes, y estamos eval-

uándolos cuidadosamente. Hemos hecho un electrocardiograma y otros estudios para obtener una imagen completa de su situación.

F: ¿Qué tipo de tratamiento va a recibir?

HP: Eso dependerá del diagnóstico final. Una vez que tengamos todos los resultados, discutiremos el plan de tratamiento con ustedes. Queremos asegurarnos de que reciba la atención adecuada y el mejor cuidado posible.

F: Gracias por su atención. Estamos asustados, pero confiamos en ustedes.

HP: Entendemos completamente sus preocupaciones. Estamos aquí para apoyarles y mantenerles informados en todo momento. Por favor, siéntanse libres de hacer cualquier pregunta o expresar cualquier inquietud que tengan. Estamos comprometidos en brindar el mejor cuidado a su ser querido.

Translation:

HP: Good morning, family. I'm Dr. Green, and we're caring for your loved one right now. I understand that you are worried but let me provide you with some important information.

F: How is she? What's going on?

HP: We understand that this is distressing. Your family member is being cared for by our medical team. We are conducting tests to determine the cause of her discomfort. Please rest assured knowing that we are doing everything we can to help her.

F: Can you tell us what is happening?

HP: Sure. Your loved one has experienced chest pain and difficulty breathing. These symptoms are concerning and we are carefully evaluating them. We have done an EKG and other tests to get a complete picture of her situation.

F: What type of treatment is she going to receive?

HP: That will depend on the final diagnosis. Once we have all the results, we will discuss the treatment plan with you. We want to make sure she receives the proper attention and the best care possible.

F: Thank you for your attention. We are scared, but we trust you.

HP: We completely understand your concerns. We are here to support you and keep you informed at all times. Please feel free to ask any questions or express any concerns you may have. We are committed to providing the best care for your loved one.

4

SPECIALIZED TERMS, TAILORED DIALOGUES

I n healthcare, communication isn't merely about language; it's about understanding and addressing the specific needs of patients in various medical contexts. Whether you're in cardiology, pediatrics, obstetrics, or any other specialized field, effective communication is the linchpin of quality care. This chapter serves as a valuable resource to help bridge language barriers and ensure the best possible outcomes for your patients.

From discussing pediatric care to explaining surgical procedures in cardiology, we will explore specialized terms and dialogues relevant to different medical fields. By the end of this chapter, you will have a comprehensive toolkit to engage with patients across a spectrum of healthcare scenarios, fostering trust, empathy, and effective communication.

Let's embark on this journey to enhance your language skills and elevate your ability to provide exceptional care in specialized areas of healthcare.

PEDIATRICS: SPEAKING SPANISH FOR THE LITTLE ONES

In this section, we delve into the nuances of pediatric care, focusing on the specialized vocabulary and empathetic dialogues that healthcare professionals should employ when dealing with young patients and their anxious parents.

One fundamental aspect of pediatric care is understanding and using specialized medical terminology effectively. For example, when discussing common childhood illnesses such as measles, you'll need to know how it translates to Spanish: *"sarampión."* This ensures that there is no room for misunderstanding, allowing for precise communication.

Parents play a crucial role in a child's healthcare journey, and effective communication with them is paramount. Employing phrases like *"Su hijo se recuperará pronto"* (Your child will recover soon) can offer comfort, hope, and a sense of assurance. These words are not only informative but also provide emotional support during challenging times.

Children can also often feel anxious or scared in a medical setting, making it essential to employ words and phrases that provide comfort and encouragement. For instance, addressing their fear of pain is vital. Utilize phrases like *"No te preocupes, esto no dolerá"* (Don't worry, this won't hurt) to alleviate their concerns when facing medical procedures.

Using positive reinforcement can significantly impact a child's experience. Simple words like "*valiente*" (brave) not only acknowledge their courage but also empower them to face medical procedures with confidence.

In the following chart, you can find some useful phrases and words to use with young patients and their parents:

Phrase	Spanish translation	Pronunciation
How are you feeling today?	*¿Cómo te sientes hoy?*	Koh-moh teh see-ehn-tehs oh-ee
You will recover soon.	*Te recuperarás pronto.*	Teh reh-koo-peh-rah-rahs prohn-toh
Don't worry, it won't hurt.	*No te preocupes, no dolerá.*	Noh teh preh-oh-koo-pehs, noh doh-leh-rah
You are very brave.	*Eres muy valiente.*	Eh-rehs moo-ee vah-lee-en-teh
We're here to help you.	*Estamos aquí para ayudarte.*	Ehs-tah-mohs ah-kee pah-rah ah-yoo-dahr-teh
It's just a small pinch.	*Es solo un pequeño piquete.*	Ehs soh-loh oon peh-keh-nyoh pee-keh-teh
This won't take long.	*Esto no tomará mucho tiempo.*	Ehs-toh noh toh-mah-rah moo-choh tee-ehm-poh
Your parents are waiting.	*Tus padres están esperando.*	Toos pah-dres ehs-tahn ehs-peh-rahn-doh
You're doing great.	*Lo estás haciendo muy bien.*	Loh ehs-tahs ah-see-ehn-doh moo-ee bee-ehn
It's okay to be scared.	*Está bien tener miedo.*	Ehs-tah bee-ehn teh-nehr mee-eh-doh

The following chart contains specific language for pediatric use:

Spanish phrase	Pronunciation	English translation
Resfriado	rehs-free-ah-doh	Cold
Fiebre	fee-eh-breh	Fever
Vacuna	bah-koo-nah	Vaccine
Varicela	vah-ree-seh-lah	Chickenpox
Asma	ahs-mah	Asthma
Dolor de garganta	doh-lohr deh gahr-GAHN-tah	Sore throat
Tos	tohs	Cough
Conjuntivitis	kohn-hoon-tee-vee-teess	Conjunctivitis (Pink eye)
Alergia	ah-lehr-hee-ah	Allergy
Fractura	frahk-too-rah	Fracture
Cirugía	see-roo-hee-ah	Surgery
Radiografía	rah-dee-oh-grah-fee-ah	X-ray
Anestesia	ah-neh-steh-see-ah	Anesthesia
Examen físico	eh-ksah-men fee-see-koh	Physical examination
Hospitalización	oh-spee-tahl-lee-sah-see-ohn	Hospitalization
Terapia física	teh-rah-pee-ah fee-see-kah	Physical therapy
Medicamento	meh-dee-kah-men-toh	Medication
Inmunización	een-moo-nee-sah-syon	Immunization
Tratamiento	trah-tah-myehn-toh	Treatment

As a footnote, I want to highlight the fact that as you can see, dear reader, some words have been repeated along the charts, like "fever" or "pain". This is due to practical reasons; I want you to use this book as a handy guide to check while you talk with your patients in different contexts.

CARDIOLOGY: DECODING THE HEART IN SPANISH

Understanding specialized medical terminology and communicating effectively with patients in the field of cardiology is crucial for accurate diagnosis and treatment. While terms like "*infarto de miocardio*" (myocardial infarction) and "*arritmia*" (arrhythmia) are specific to this field, it's essential to use simple language when discussing complex conditions with Spanish-speaking patients. For instance, using phrases like "*problema del corazón*" (heart problem) can help patients comprehend their condition more quickly.

Moreover, explaining procedures in Spanish can enhance patient comfort and cooperation. Phrases such as "*Vamos a hacer un electrocardiograma*" (We are going to do an EKG) can prepare patients for upcoming tests or examinations, ensuring they are at ease throughout their medical experience.

So, from the following chart, you can learn specific vocabulary associated with this field of medical care, beginning with the most common diseases and cardiovascular affections, ordered alphabetically for practical purposes:

English term	Spanish translation	Pronunciation
Angina	Angina	ahn-hee-nah
Aortic Aneurysm	Aneurisma aórtico	ah-neh-oo-reez-mah ah-ohr-tee-koh
Arrhythmia	Arritmia	ah-reet-mee-ah
Atherosclerosis	Aterosclerosis	ah-teh-rohs-kleh-roh-sis
Cardiac Arrest	Paro cardíaco	pah-roh kahr-dee-ah-koh
Chest Pain	Dolor en el pecho	doh-lohr en el peh-choh
Congenital Heart Defect	Defecto cardíaco congénito	deh-fehk-toh kahr-dee-ah-koh kohn-heh-nee-toh
Coronary Artery Disease	Enfermedad de las arterias coronarias	ehn-fehr-meh-dah deh lahs ahr-teh-ree-ahs koh-roh-nah-ree-ahs
Heart Attack	Ataque al corazón	ah-tah-keh ahl koh-rah-sohn
Heart Disease	Enfermedad cardíaca	ehn-fehr-meh-dah kahr-dee-ah-kah
High Blood Pressure	Presión arterial alta	preh-see-ohn ahr-teh-ree-ahl ahl-tah
Myocardial Infarction	Infarto de miocardio	een-fahr-toh deh mee-oh-kahr-dee-oh
Palpitations	Palpitaciones	pahl-pee-tah-see-oh-nehs
Stroke	Derrame cerebral	deh-rah-meh seh-reh-brahl
Valve Disease	Enfermedad de la válvula	ehn-fehr-meh-dah deh lah vahl-voo-lah

In the following one, you'll find the most common medical procedures, sorted by the same criteria:

English term	Spanish translation	Pronunciation
Angioplasty	Angioplastia	an-hee-oh-plahs-tee-ah
Cardiac Catheterization	Cateterismo Cardíaco	kah-teh-teh-reez-moh kahr-dee-ah-koh
Coronary Artery Bypass Surgery	Cirugía de Bypass de Arterias Coronarias	see-roo-hee-ah deh bye-pass deh ar-teh-ree-ahs koh-roh-nah-ree-ahs
Defibrillation	Desfibrilación	des-fee-bree-lah-syon
Echocardiogram	Ecocardiograma	eh-koh-kahr-dee-oh-gram-ah
Heart Transplant	Trasplante de Corazón	trahs-plan-teh deh koh-rah-sohn
Pacemaker	Marcapasos	mahr-kah-pah-sohs
Stent	Stent	stent
Treadmill Stress Test	Prueba de Esfuerzo en Cinta	prwoo-eh-bah deh ehs-fwehr-soh ehn seen-tah
Valve Replacement Surgery	Cirugía de Reemplazo de Válvula	see-roo-hee-ah deh reh-em-plah-soh deh vahl-voo-lah

NEUROLOGY: NAVIGATING THE BRAIN IN SPANISH

Now it's time to address the proper technical language to communicate with Spanish speakers about their neurological health. Below, you will find some of the most common terms for health issues and treatments:

English term	Spanish translation	Pronunciation
Alzheimer's Disease	*Enfermedad de Alzheimer*	en-fehr-meh-dah deh ahlz-hai-mer
Brain Tumor	*Tumor Cerebral*	too-mohr seh-reh-brahl
Epilepsy	*Epilepsia*	eh-pee-lep-see-ah
Migraine	*Migraña*	mee-grah-nyah
Parkinson's Disease	*Enfermedad de Parkinson*	en-fehr-meh-dah deh pahr-khin-sawn
Seizure	*Convulsión*	kohn-vool-see-own
Synapse	*Sinapsis*	see-nahp-sees
Nervous System	*Sistema Nervioso*	see-steh-mah nehr-vee-oh-soh
Memory Loss	*Pérdida de Memoria*	pehr-dee-dah deh meh-moh-ree-ah
Brain Surgery	*Cirugía Cerebral*	see-roo-hee-ah seh-reh-brahl
EEG (Electroencephalogram)	*EEG (Electroencefalograma)*	ee-ee-gee (eh-lehk-troh-ehn-seh-fah-loh-grah-mah)
Neurological Examination	*Examen Neurológico*	ehk-sah-men nehw-roh-loh-hee-koh
Lumbar Puncture	*Punción Lumbar*	poon-see-ohn loom-bahr
MRI (Magnetic Resonance Imaging)	*Resonancia Magnética*	reh-soh-nahn-see-ah mahg-neh-tee-kah

Brain Scan	Tomografía Cerebral	toh-moh-grah-fee-ah seh-reh-brahl
Physical Therapy	Terapia Física	teh-rah-pee-ah fee-see-kah
Nerve Block	Bloqueo Nervioso	bloh-keh-oh nehr-vee-oh-soh
Deep Brain Stimulation	Estimulación Profunda Cerebral	eh-stee-moo-lah-syon proh-foon-dah seh-reh-brahl
Neurotransmitter Replacement	Reemplazo de Neurotransmisores	reh-ehm-plah-soh deh neh-oo-roh-trahns-mee-soh-rehs

ONCOLOGY: EXPLAINING CANCER CARE IN SPANISH

In the field of oncology, sensitivity in language is of paramount importance due to the delicate nature of cancer care. Patients facing cancer need not only medical explanations but also emotional support.

This medical field comprises a wide array of specific terminologies, ranging from types of cancer to various treatment options. Common terms in this field include "quimioterapia" (chemotherapy) and "radioterapia" (radiation therapy). When explaining these terms in Spanish, it's crucial to do so with sensitivity and care. Instead of using complex medical jargon, it's often more comforting to describe treatments as "tratamiento para combatir el cáncer" (treatment to fight cancer), emphasizing the goal of the intervention.

Beyond the medical aspects, supporting a cancer patient in Spanish involves providing emotional support and reassurance. Phrases like "Estamos contigo en cada paso del camino" (We are with you every step of the way) can convey a sense of companionship and comfort during what can be a challenging journey.

Let's address the necessary vocabulary to communicate with patients:

Cancer diseases and conditions

English term	Spanish translation	Pronunciation
Lung Cancer	*Cáncer de Pulmón*	kahn-sehr deh pool-mohn
Breast Cancer	*Cáncer de Mama*	kahn-sehr deh mah-mah
Prostate Cancer	*Cáncer de Próstata*	kahn-sehr deh proh-stah-tah
Leukemia	*Leucemia*	leh-oo-seh-mee-ah
Lymphoma	*Linfoma*	leen-foh-mah
Skin Cancer	*Cáncer de Piel*	kahn-sehr deh pee-ehl
Brain Tumor	*Tumor Cerebral*	too-mohr seh-reh-brahl
Colon Cancer	*Cáncer de Colon*	kahn-sehr deh koh-lon
Ovarian Cancer	*Cáncer de Ovario*	kahn-sehr deh oh-vah-ree-oh
Pancreatic Cancer	*Cáncer de Páncreas*	kahn-sehr deh pahn-kree-ahs
Bladder Cancer	*Cáncer de Vejiga*	kahn-sehr deh veh-hee-gah
Cervical Cancer	*Cáncer Cervical*	kahn-sehr sehr-vee-kahl
Testicular Cancer	*Cáncer Testicular*	kahn-sehr tes-tee-koo-lahr
Thyroid Cancer	*Cáncer de Tiroides*	kahn-sehr deh tee-roy-dehs
Bone Cancer	*Cáncer de Huesos*	kahn-sehr deh weh-sohs

Medical procedures and treatments:

English term	Spanish translation	Pronunciation
Chemotherapy	Quimioterapia	kee-mee-oh-teh-rah-pee-ah
Radiation Therapy	Radioterapia	rah-dee-oh-teh-rah-pee-ah
Surgery	Cirugía	see-roo-hee-ah
Biopsy	Biopsia	bee-op-see-ah
Immunotherapy	Inmunoterapia	een-moo-noh-teh-rah-pee-ah
Targeted Therapy	Terapia Dirigida	teh-rah-pee-ah dee-ree-hee-dah
Stem Cell Transplant	Trasplante de Células Madre	trahs-plan-teh deh seh-loo-lahs mah-dreh
Hormone Therapy	Terapia Hormonal	teh-rah-pee-ah hohr-moh-nahl
Palliative Care	Cuidados Paliativos	kwee-dah-dohs pah-lee-ah-tee-vohs
Genetic Testing	Pruebas Genéticas	prooeh-bahs heh-neh-tee-kahs
Radiosurgery	Radiocirugía	rah-dee-oh-see-roo-hee-ah
Bone Marrow Transplant	Trasplante de Médula Ósea	trahs-plan-teh deh meh-doo-lah oh-seh-ah
Ultrasound	Ecografía	eh-koh-grah-fee-ah
Blood Transfusion	Transfusión de Sangre	trahns-foo-see-ohn deh sahn-greh

Clinical Trials	Ensayos Clínicos	ehn-sah-yohs klee-nee-kohs
Radiation Oncology	Oncología Radioterápica	on-koh-loh-hee-ah rah-dee-oh-teh-rah-pee-kah
Mammogram	Mamografía	mah-moh-grah-fee-ah
Chemoradiation	Quimiorradiación	kee-mee-oh-rah-dee-ah-see-ohn
Supportive Care	Cuidados de Soporte	kwee-dah-dohs deh soh-pohr-teh

EXERCISES AND PRACTICE

A. Read the following story and answer the questions:

Había una vez una enfermera llamada Marta que trabajaba en un hospital pediátrico. Un día, le asignaron la tarea de cuidar a Sofía, una niña de cinco años que había sido diagnosticada con varicela y también tenía un resfriado común. Sofía estaba muy asustada porque tenía muchas manchas rojas en su piel y sentía picazón por todo el cuerpo. Además, sabía que tendría que recibir algunas vacunas y tratamientos para aliviar sus síntomas.

Marta entró en la habitación de Sofía con una sonrisa cálida y le dijo: "¡Hola, Sofía! Soy Marta, tu enfermera hoy. Estoy aquí para cuidarte y asegurarme de que te sientas mejor pronto". Sofía miró a Marta con ojos preocupados y preguntó: "¿Me va a picar mucho cuando me pongan las inyecciones?".

Marta se agachó a la altura de Sofía y le explicó con ternura: "Sé que las inyecciones pueden asustar un poco, pero te prometo que serán rápidas y que estaré contigo todo el tiempo. También te traeré algo para la picazón en la piel". Sofía asintió con cautela, pareciendo un poco más tranquila.

Durante el día, Marta cuidó de Sofía, le dio medicamentos para aliviar su resfriado y aplicó loción calmante en sus manchas de varicela. También le trajo algunos libros para colorear y jugar juntas. Marta hizo todo lo posible para que Sofía se sintiera cómoda y segura.

Al final del día, Sofía sonrió y le dijo a Marta: "Gracias, enfermera Marta. No fue tan malo como pensaba. ¡Me siento mejor ahora!". Marta le acarició el cabello y respondió: "Estoy feliz de que te sientas mejor, Sofía. Siempre estamos aquí para cuidarte y hacer que te sientas lo más cómoda possible".

Questions:

1. Who is Sofia?_____
2. What were her symptoms?

   _____

3. What was she afraid of?

   _____

4. How did Marta manage it?

   _____

Translation:

Once upon a time, there was a nurse named Marta who worked in a pediatric hospital. One day, she was assigned the task of taking care of Sofia, a five-year-old girl who had been diagnosed with chickenpox and also had a common cold. Sofia was very scared because she had many red spots on her skin and she felt itchy all over her body. Additionally, she knew that she would have to receive some vaccines and treatments to alleviate her symptoms.

Marta entered Sofía's room with a warm smile and said, "Hello, Sofía! I'm Marta, your nurse today. I'm here to take care of you and make sure you feel better soon." Sofia looked at Marta with worried eyes and asked, "Will I be really itchy when they give me the injections?"

Marta crouched down to Sofia's height and explained tenderly: "I know the injections can be a little scary, but I promise they will be quick and that I will be with you the entire time. I will also bring you something for your itchy skin." Sofia nodded cautiously, seeming a little calmer.

During the day, Marta took care of Sofía, giving her medicine to relieve her cold and applying soothing lotion to her chickenpox spots. She also brought her some books to color and play with together. Marta did everything possible to make Sofía feel comfortable and safe.

At the end of the day, Sofia smiled and said to Marta, "Thank you, Nurse Marta. It wasn't as bad as she thought. I feel better now!" Marta stroked her hair and responded, "I'm happy that you feel better, Sofía. We are always here to take care of you and make you feel as comfortable as possible."

B. Complete the following sentences:

1. *Durante la _____ cardíaca, se registraron anormalidades en el ECG.*
2. *La cirugía de bypass coronario es un tratamiento común para la _____.*
3. *El marcapasos es un dispositivo utilizado para regular el ritmo _____.*
4. *El electrocardiograma es una prueba que registra la actividad _____.*
5. *El infarto de miocardio se produce cuando hay un bloqueo en una arteria _____.*
6. *La _____ puede causar dificultad para respirar y fatiga.*
7. *El paciente se sometió a un cateterismo cardíaco para evaluar la salud de sus _____.*
8. *La _____ cardíaca puede deberse a la acumulación de placa en las arterias.*
9. *La angina de pecho es un síntoma de que el corazón no recibe suficiente _____.*

Answers:

1. *Arritmia*
2. *Enfermedad cardíaca coronaria*
3. *Cardíaco*
4. *Cardíaca*
5. *Coronaria*
6. *Insuficiencia cardíaca*
7. *Arterias coronarias*

8. *Enfermedad*

9. *Oxígeno*

C. Read the following text. It's an abstract for a fictitious research. Then, read the translation:

Exploración de las **Alteraciones Neuromotoras** *en Pacientes con* **Esclerosis Múltiple** *mediante* **Resonancia Magnética Funcional**

Resumen:

La **esclerosis múltiple** *(EM) es una enfermedad neurológica crónica que afecta a un número significativo de individuos en todo el mundo. Uno de los aspectos más debilitantes de la EM es la aparición de* **alteraciones neuromotoras**, *que pueden limitar considerablemente la movilidad y la calidad de vida de los pacientes. En este estudio, se utilizó la* **resonancia magnética funcional** *(RMf) para investigar las bases neurobiológicas de estas alteraciones en pacientes con EM. Se reclutaron veinte pacientes diagnosticados con EM y veinte partici-pantes sanos como grupo de control. Se realizaron análisis de RMf mientras los participantes realizaban tareas motoras específicas. Los resultados revelaron* **anomalías en la conectividad funcional** *en regiones cerebrales clave involucradas en el control motor en los pacientes con EM en comparación con el grupo de control. Estos hallazgos proporcionan una comprensión más profunda de las* **alteraciones neuromotoras** *en la EM y pueden tener implicaciones importantes para el desarrollo de terapias dirigidas a mejorar la función motora en esta población de pacientes.*

Translation:

Exploration of Neuromotor Alterations in Patients with Multiple Sclerosis through Functional Magnetic Resonance Imaging

Abstract:

Multiple sclerosis (MS) is a chronic neurological disease that affects a significant number of individuals worldwide. One of the most debilitating aspects of MS is the onset of neuromotor alterations, which can significantly limit mobility and the quality of life for patients. In this study, functional magnetic resonance imaging (fMRI) was used to investigate the neurobiological basis of these alterations in patients with MS. Twenty patients diagnosed with MS and, as a control group, twenty healthy participants were recruited. fMRI analyses were conducted while participants performed specific motor tasks. The results revealed abnormalities in functional connectivity in key brain regions involved in motor control in MS patients compared to the control group. These findings provide a deeper understanding of neuromotor alterations in MS and may have important implications for the development of therapies aimed at improving motor function in this patient population.

D. Read the following conversation and complete the translation below:

HP: Buenas tardes, ¿cómo se encuentra hoy?

P: Buenas tardes, doctor. Me siento muy nerviosa y asustada.

HP: Entiendo que esto puede ser abrumador. Hemos realizado algunas pruebas y quiero hablarle sobre los resultados. Hemos detectado un tumor mamario, y es importante que comencemos el tratamiento de inmediato para evitar que se propague.

P: ¿Un tumor? ¿Qué significa eso? ¿Es cáncer?

HP: Sí, es un tumor en la mama, y debemos tratarlo con seriedad. La buena noticia es que lo hemos detectado a tiempo, y eso es crucial para el tratamiento. Quiero que sepa que estamos aquí para apoyarla en cada paso del camino.

P: ¿Qué vamos a hacer ahora?

HP: Lo primero que haremos es realizar más pruebas para determinar el tipo exacto de tumor y su extensión. Luego, trabajaremos juntos para desarrollar un plan de tratamiento personalizado que podría incluir cirugía, quimioterapia o radioterapia, dependiendo de lo que sea mejor para usted.

P: ¿Cuánto tiempo llevará el tratamiento? ¿Será doloroso?

HP: El tiempo de tratamiento varía según su caso, y trabajaremos para hacerlo lo más cómodo posible. Algunos aspectos pueden causar molestias, pero estaremos aquí para manejar cualquier síntoma que pueda experimentar. Su bienestar es nuestra principal preocupación.

P: Gracias, doctor, por ser comprensivo. Esto es aterrador, pero sé que estoy en buenas manos.

HP: Estamos aquí para usted, y juntos superaremos esto. Estaremos con usted en cada paso del camino y haremos todo lo posible para brindarle el mejor cuidado.

Translation:

HP: Good afternoon. How are you feeling today?

P: Good afternoon, doctor. I'm feeling very nervous and scared.

HP: I understand that this can be overwhelming. We have conducted some tests and I want to talk to you about the results. We have detected a _____ (1), and it's important to start treatment immediately to prevent it from spreading.

P: A tumor? What does that mean? Is it _____(2)?

HP: Yes, it's a tumor in the breast, and we must take it seriously. The good news is that we have detected it in time and that is crucial for treatment. I want you to know that we are here to support you every step of the way.

P: What are we going to do now?

HP: The first thing we will do is perform more tests to determine the exact type of tumor and its extent. Then, we will work together to develop a personalized treatment plan that could include surgery, _____ (3), or _____ (4), depending on what is best for you.

P: How long will the treatment take? Will it be _____ (5)?

HP: The treatment time varies depending on your case, and we will work to make it as comfortable as possible. Some aspects may cause discomfort, but we will be here to manage any symptoms you may experience. Your well-being is our top concern.

P: Thank you, doctor, for being understanding. This is terrifying, but I know I'm in good hands.

HP: We are here for you, and together we will overcome this. We will be with you every step of the way and do everything we can to provide you with the best care.

Answers:

1. Breast tumor
2. Cancer
3. Chemotherapy
4. Radiation therapy
5. Painful

CROSSING THE CULTURAL BRIDGE: SENSITIVITY IN SPANISH-SPEAKING PATIENT CARE

Effective communication in healthcare goes beyond language proficiency. It encompasses cultural awareness and sensitivity, recognizing that each patient brings a unique cultural background and perspective. This is especially evident when delivering care to Spanish-speaking patients and their families. While speaking Spanish is crucial, it's just the beginning. Understanding and respecting cultural subtleties can make a significant difference in offering patient-centered, empathetic care.

Spanish-speaking patients often come from diverse backgrounds, representing a rich variety of cultures and traditions. As healthcare professionals, your responsibility extends beyond addressing physical symptoms. It involves acknowledging and honoring the values, beliefs, and customs that influence the patient's worldview. Neglecting this cultural bridge can result in misunderstandings, hinder trust-building, and ultimately impact the quality of care.

Picture a scenario where a healthcare provider, despite being fluent in Spanish, unintentionally offends a patient by not recognizing the significance of family in their culture. Or envision a situation where a doctor prescribes treatment without considering the patient's cultural preferences and dietary restrictions, leading to non-compliance and adverse outcomes. These are just a few instances that illustrate the intricate relationship between language and culture in healthcare.

In this chapter, we will explore the cultural intricacies of Spanish-speaking patients and offer practical insights to healthcare professionals. These insights aim to ensure sensitivity and patient-focused care. By doing so, we aim to bridge the gap between language and culture, cultivating an atmosphere of trust and understanding that enriches the healthcare experience for both providers and patients.

EMBRACING CULTURAL DIVERSITY IN HEALTHCARE

Hospitals, clinics, and healthcare facilities across the globe serve a wide array of patients from various cultural backgrounds. While this diversity can indeed present challenges, it also provides an opportunity to enrich our understanding of health and wellness from different perspectives.

Studies have consistently demonstrated the profound impact of cultural sensitivity on healthcare outcomes (Krist et al., 2017). Patients who feel understood and respected by their healthcare providers are more likely to adhere to treatment plans, leading to improved health results. The converse is equally true; a lack of cultural awareness can lead to misunderstandings, patient dissatisfaction, and compromised treatment effectiveness.

One of the key takeaways from this is that a healthcare professional's ability to navigate and comprehend cultural nuances is more than just a diplomatic gesture; it is an essential aspect of delivering high-quality care. Understanding a patient's cultural background can make a significant difference in building trust and fostering effective communication.

Let's delve into a concrete example. Many Hispanic cultures have deep-rooted beliefs in holistic and natural medicine, often passed down through generations. Recognizing and respecting these beliefs is essential for healthcare professionals. It means being open to discussions about treatment options that align with these beliefs, or at the very least, acknowledging their significance in the patient's overall well-being.

For instance, a patient might express a preference for traditional herbal remedies alongside conventional medical treatment. A healthcare provider who is aware of and sensitive to these cultural preferences can engage in a productive conversation, exploring the compatibility of traditional and modern approaches to healthcare. This level of understanding goes a long way in fostering patient trust, satisfaction, and ultimately, better health outcomes.

306 | SOL MANCILLA

Let the following stories be examples of how these cultural barriers can look in real-life scenarios:

- Imagine a Spanish-speaking patient, Maria, visiting a hospital for a critical consultation. The healthcare provider primarily speaks English and relies on an interpreter to communicate with Maria. While the interpreter does their best, subtle nuances and emotions in Maria's speech may be lost in translation. This gap in direct communication can lead to misunderstandings and hinder the provider's ability to fully comprehend Maria's symptoms and concerns. Moreover, Maria may feel frustrated or anxious due to her inability to express herself directly, impacting her overall experience and trust in the healthcare system.
- Juan, a Hispanic patient, has been diagnosed with a chronic illness. He believes strongly in the healing properties of herbal remedies passed down through his family for generations. When his healthcare provider suggests a treatment plan that solely relies on pharmaceutical medications, Juan feels misunderstood and resistant to the proposed approach. The provider, unaware of Juan's cultural beliefs, struggles to convince him of the benefits of modern medicine. This disconnect in understanding may lead to Juan seeking alternative treatments independently, potentially compromising his health.

These scenarios illustrate how cultural barriers, such as language differences and a lack of awareness about patients' cultural beliefs, can manifest in real-life healthcare interactions. Effective cultural competence training and open communication can help healthcare professionals overcome these barriers and provide more patient-centered care.

COMMON BELIEFS AND CUSTOMS IN SPANISH-SPEAKING CULTURES

Understanding and respecting the common beliefs and customs prevalent in Spanish-speaking cultures is vital for healthcare professionals aiming to provide culturally sensitive care. These beliefs and customs influence various aspects of patient care and can significantly impact patient satisfaction and treatment outcomes.

In many Spanish-speaking cultures, the family unit plays a central role in a person's life, including healthcare decisions. It's common for patients to involve multiple family members in discussions about their health and treatment options. Healthcare professionals should be prepared to accommodate and engage with extended family members who may accompany the patient to medical appointments. Understanding that family support is highly valued can enhance the patient-provider relationship.

Example: Carmen, a Mexican-American patient, brings her parents and siblings to her prenatal check-up. The obstetrician acknowledges and welcomes the family's presence, fostering a supportive environment.

Magical or supernatural beliefs may be a common component to mind, especially when treating older patients. The concept of "*susto*" or "fright sickness" is prevalent in many Hispanic cultures. It is believed that a sudden scare or traumatic experience can lead to physical and emotional distress. Healthcare professionals should recognize that patients may attribute their symptoms to such experiences. Understanding "*susto*" can help providers empathize with patients' concerns and respectfully explain medical conditions with their cultural beliefs.

Example: A patient, Javier, presents with unexplained anxiety and physical symptoms after witnessing a traumatic event. His therapist acknowledges the possibility of "*susto*" and incorporates trauma-informed care into the treatment plan.

On the other hand, we must address gender matters to deeply understand the Hispanic communicational dynamics. When it comes to treating Hispanic men, it's important to be aware of their cultural nuances when seeking medical advice.

"*Machismo*" refers to the traditional cultural expectation that men should be strong, stoic, and unemotional. This view influences how men perceive and express their health concerns. Men might be more reluctant to seek medical help or admit vulnerability. Healthcare professionals should be proactive in asking about symptoms and offering support, creating a safe space for male patients to discuss their health.

Example: Carlos, a Hispanic patient, experiences persistent chest pain but hesitates to seek medical attention due to the fear of appearing weak. His cardiologist engages in open dialogue, assuring him that seeking help is a sign of strength and responsibility.

Understanding and respecting these cultural nuances can bridge the gap between healthcare professionals and Spanish-speaking patients, fostering trust, effective communication, and improved healthcare outcomes.

As I previously mentioned, treating Hispanic people has its specific challenges, since their cultural background plays a role when it comes to health care. The following tips will help you navigate successfully these situations:

- Using the **patient's last name** with an appropriate title (Mr., Mrs., etc.) is a sign of respect, particularly when addressing older individuals. It acknowledges their life experience and dignity.
- Non-verbal communication, including gestures, can vary in meaning across cultures. **Being cautious with gestures** ensures that no unintended offense is taken due to cultural differences.
- It's essential to assess the clarity and cultural sensitivity of questions and instructions. **Avoid assumptions** and be prepared to **rephrase** or **provide additional context** when necessary.
- Encouraging patients to **ask questions** fosters open and transparent communication. Many patients may have concerns or require clarification but may hesitate to speak up unless prompted.
- Relying on children to translate can create awkward power dynamics within the family and may not ensure

accurate communication. If the situation demands it, it's best to use professional interpreters or language services to maintain confidentiality and accuracy.

- Be conscious of **body language** and physical contact norms. While some Hispanic cultures may have a preference for standing closer to each other while talking and using physical touch as a sign of warmth, this may not always be appropriate in a professional healthcare setting. Strike a balance between showing empathy and respecting personal and professional boundaries.

These recommendations reflect a commitment to patient-centered care and cultural competence. Healthcare professionals who follow these guidelines can enhance the patient experience and build trust with their Hispanic patients and patients from diverse backgrounds.

OVERCOMING CULTURAL BARRIERS: CASE STUDIES AND EXAMPLES

The ability to overcome cultural barriers in healthcare is a skill that healthcare professionals develop over time. Real-life case studies and examples provide valuable insights into the nuances of cultural sensitivity and how it can positively impact patient care. Here are two illustrative examples:

Imagine a Bolivian patient who attributes their illness to "*mal de ojo*" or the "evil eye," a common belief in many Hispanic cultures. Rather than dismissing this belief as superstition, a culturally sensitive healthcare professional might acknowledge the patient's concerns. They can then explain how medical treatments can be viewed as tools to "fight" the evil eye, aligning the patient's cultural belief with Western medical interventions. This approach helps the patient feel understood and respected, fostering trust and compliance with treatment recommendations.

Now, consider another scenario where a Mexican patient is diagnosed with diabetes. As traditional foods hold significant cultural and social importance in Mexican family life, instead of advising the patient to eliminate these foods entirely, a culturally sensitive approach involves discussing portion control and healthier cooking methods. The healthcare professional can work collaboratively with the patient to adapt traditional recipes to meet dietary requirements, ensuring that cultural customs remain untouched while promoting better health outcomes.

These examples emphasize the significance of understanding and respecting cultural nuances in healthcare.

Just as mastering medical vocabulary and verbal tenses is crucial, understanding and respecting cultural beliefs and customs play an indispensable role in providing effective and empathetic care, especially when treating Hispanic patients.

Our journey through cultural sensitivity has highlighted the importance of showing respect, asking questions, and being adaptable in our approach to care. We've learned that small gestures, like addressing patients by their preferred names or maintaining eye contact, can make a significant difference in building trust and rapport. We've seen that involving family members in healthcare decisions and being aware of patients' beliefs about health and illness contribute to a more patient-centered and culturally sensitive practice.

EXERCISES AND PRACTICE

A. Read the following text and answer—in Spanish—the questions below:

Me mudé a los Estados Unidos con mi hijo para estar más cerca de él y de mis nietos. Dejar mi país natal, Perú, no fue fácil; significaba dejar atrás la familiaridad de mi entorno, a mis amigos y todo lo que había conocido durante la mayor parte de mi vida. Pero la familia era mi ancla, y quería estar cerca de ellos. No sabía que este viaje me llevaría a un encuentro inesperado con la atención médica en tierras extranjeras.

A medida que pasaban los años, me adapté a mi nueva vida, pero algo no estaba bien. Un persistente y molesto dolor en la espalda comenzó a afligirme. Intenté descartarlo como el resultado natural del envejecimiento, como otros sugerían, o el resultado de una mala postura. Sin embargo, en lo más profundo de mí, sabía que había algo más en ello.

Mi hijo y mis nietos hicieron todo lo posible por cuidarme, instándome a buscar consejo médico. Estaban genuinamente preocupados por mi salud, pero yo vacilaba. Siempre había sido la que ofrecía consuelo y fuerza a mi familia, y la idea de cargarlos con mi dolor me resultaba insoportable.

Lo que no entendían era que este dolor, este peso invisible que parecía estar doblando mi espalda, era más que una dolencia física. Era el reflejo de un secreto familiar guardado durante mucho tiempo, un silencio que había llevado desde mi juventud. Sabía que este silencio, esta verdad no dicha, estaba en la raíz de mi sufrimiento.

Visitaba a varios médicos que, a pesar de sus mejores intenciones, no podían comprender la profundidad de mi angustia. Me hicieron pruebas, me sugirieron medicamentos y hasta me recomendaron fisioterapia, pero no los escuché, porque sabía—o pensaba—que ninguna de esas cosas podía aliviar mi dolor.

Entonces, un día, mientras el dolor me inmovilizaba y la desesperación amenazaba con consumirme, apareció un rayo de esperanza. Conocí al Dr. Rodríguez, un médico mexicano-americano que practicaba la medicina con una mezcla única de conocimiento occidental y sensibilidad cultural. Cuando compartí mi creencia de que mi dolor de espalda estaba relacionado con este secreto oculto, él no lo descartó ni me trató con condescendencia. En cambio, me escuchó atentamente, validando mis experiencias y emociones.

El Dr. Rodríguez reconoció que mi bienestar físico y emocional estaban entrelazados. Recomendó una cirugía de espalda para abordar el aspecto físico de mi sufrimiento y sugirió que hablara con un consejero para liberarme del secreto familiar que me había atormentado durante tanto tiempo.

Bajo el cuidado del Dr. Rodríguez, me sometí a la cirugía necesaria y, aunque la recuperación fue desafiante, mi dolor de espalda se fue reduciendo gradualmente. Al mismo tiempo, comencé mis sesiones con un consejero, desenredando el secreto arraigado que me había cargado durante décadas. No fue un viaje fácil, pero con el apoyo del Dr. Rodríguez y la orientación de mi consejero, sentí que finalmente se estaba levantando un peso pesado.

Hoy, me mantengo un poco más erguida, no solo físicamente sino también emocionalmente. He aprendido la importancia de los profesionales de la salud que no solo tratan el cuerpo, sino que también reconocen la compleja interacción entre la salud física y emocional. El enfoque compasivo y culturalmente sensible del Dr. Rodríguez me mostró el poder de la comprensión y la validación en el proceso de curación.

Translation:

I moved to the United States with my son to be closer to him and my grandchildren. Leaving my home country of Peru was not easy; it meant leaving behind the familiarity of my surroundings, my friends, and everything I had known for most of my life. But family was my anchor, and I wanted to be near them. Little did I know that this journey would lead me to an unexpected encounter with healthcare in a foreign land.

As the years passed, I settled into my new life, but something was amiss. A persistent, gnawing pain in my back began to afflict me. I tried to dismiss it as the natural result of aging, as others suggested, or the result of poor posture. However, deep down, I knew there was something more to it.

My son and my grandchildren did their best to care for me, urging me to seek medical advice. They were genuinely concerned about my health, but I hesitated. I had always been the one to offer solace and strength to my family, and the thought of burdening them with my pain felt unbearable.

What they didn't understand was that this pain, this invisible weight that seemed to be bending my back, was more than just a physical ailment. It was a reflection of a long-held family secret, a silence that I had carried since my youth. I knew that this silence, this unspoken truth, was at the root of my suffering.

I visited various doctors who, despite their best intentions, couldn't comprehend the depth of my distress. They ran tests, suggested medications, and even recommended physical therapy, but I didn't listen to them, since I knew—or thought—none of those things were able to alleviate my pain.

Then, one day, as the pain immobilized me and despair threatened to engulf me, a ray of hope appeared. I met Dr. Rodriguez, a Mexican-American doctor who practiced medicine with a unique blend of Western knowledge and cultural sensitivity. When I shared my belief that my back pain was linked to this hidden secret, he didn't dismiss it or patronize me. Instead, he listened attentively, validating my experiences and emotions.

Dr. Rodriguez recognized that my physical and emotional well-being were intertwined. He recommended back surgery to address the physical aspect of my suffering and suggested that I speak with a counselor to unburden myself of the family secret that had plagued me for so long.

Under Dr. Rodriguez's care, I underwent the necessary surgery, and though the recovery was challenging, my back pain gradually subsided. Simultaneously, I began my sessions with a counselor, unraveling the deep-rooted secret that had weighed me down for decades. It was not an easy journey, but with Dr. Rodriguez's support and the guidance of my counselor, I felt like a heavy burden was finally being lifted.

Today, I stand a little taller, not just physically but emotionally as well. I have learned the importance of healthcare professionals who not only treat the body but also recognize the complex interplay between physical and emotional health. Dr. Rodriguez's compassionate and culturally sensitive approach showed me the power of understanding and validation in the healing process.

Questions:

1. How did the protagonist's cultural background influence her reluctance to seek medical intervention?
    _____
    _____

2. What role did the Mexican-American doctor play in addressing the protagonist's health concerns?
    _____
    _____

3. In what ways did the healthcare professionals in the story demonstrate cultural sensitivity in their approach to the patient's care?
    _____
    _____

4. What were some of the cultural barriers the protagonist faced in the healthcare system?
    _____
    _____

5. How did the healthcare professionals validate the protagonist's health beliefs and experiences?
    _____
    _____

6. What was the connection between the protagonist's physical pain and her hidden family secret, as portrayed in the story?
    _____
    _____

7. What lesson can healthcare providers learn from this narrative about the importance of culturally sensitive care and communication?
    _____
    _____

Answers:

1. *La cultura de la protagonista influyó en su renuencia a buscar intervención médica, ya que tenía creencias arraigadas sobre el dolor de espalda y su relación con un secreto de familia.*
2. *El doctor mexico-americano desempeñó un papel fundamental al escuchar y validar las creencias de salud de la protagonista. Además, la convenció de someterse a una cirugía de espalda necesaria y buscar asesoramiento para liberarse del peso de su secreto familiar.*
3. *Los profesionales de la salud en la historia demostraron sensibilidad cultural al respetar y comprender las creencias de salud de la paciente, en lugar de descartarlas.*
4. *La protagonista enfrentó barreras culturales en el sistema de atención médica cuando otros médicos intentaron convencerla de que sus creencias estaban equivocadas y que su dolor de espalda tenía otras causas.*
5. *Los profesionales de la salud validaron las creencias y experiencias de salud de la protagonista al reconocer que su dolor de espalda estaba relacionado con su secreto familiar y al ofrecer soluciones que se alineaban con sus creencias.*
6. *La conexión entre el dolor físico de la protagonista y su secreto familiar radicaba en la creencia de que guardar el secreto estaba causando el dolor. La liberación del secreto a través del asesoramiento se consideró una parte crucial de su proceso de curación.*
7. *La lección que los proveedores de atención médica pueden aprender de esta narrativa es la importancia de brindar atención y comunicación culturalmente sensibles. Es vital escuchar y respetar las creencias y experiencias de salud de los*

pacientes para proporcionar un cuidado más efectivo y compasivo.

Answers Translation:

1. The protagonist's culture influenced her reluctance to seek medical intervention, as she had deep-rooted beliefs about back pain and its relationship to a family secret.
2. The Mexican-American doctor played a key role in listening to and validating the protagonist's health beliefs. Additionally, he convinced her to undergo necessary back surgery and seek counseling to free herself from the weight of her family secret.
3. Health professionals in the story demonstrated cultural sensitivity by respecting and understanding the patient's health beliefs, rather than dismissing them.
4. The protagonist faced cultural barriers in the health care system when other doctors tried to convince her that her beliefs were wrong and that her back pain had other causes.
5. The health professionals validated the protagonist's health beliefs and experiences by recognizing that her back pain was related to her family history and by offering solutions that aligned with her beliefs.
6. The connection between the protagonist's physical pain and her family's secret lies in the belief that keeping the secret was causing the pain. Releasing the secret through her counseling was considered a crucial part of her healing process.

7. The lesson healthcare providers can learn from this narrative is the importance of providing culturally sensitive care and communication. It is vital to listen to and respect patients' health beliefs and experiences to provide more effective and compassionate care.

6

MASTERING THE INTRICACIES OF MEDICAL SPANISH

This chapter takes us deeper into the world of medical Spanish, where mastery of intricate grammar rules and complex medical terminologies becomes essential. This chapter is designed to equip healthcare professionals with the advanced language skills required to navigate intricate medical scenarios, ensuring accurate communication with Spanish-speaking patients. From the intricacies of grammar to the precision of medical terminology, the following pages provide practical insights and guidance for those committed to delivering the highest level of care to their diverse patient populations.

¡Vamos a ello!

ESCALATING YOUR GRAMMAR: THE SUBJUNCTIVE MOOD

The Spanish language is renowned for its rich grammatical features, and one of the most intricate aspects is the subjunctive mood. In medical contexts, understanding and utilizing the subjunctive mood is vital for healthcare professionals seeking to communicate with precision and nuance. This mood is often employed to express various states of unreality, including doubt, possibility, necessity, and actions that have not yet occurred. Let's delve into how the subjunctive mood functions in Spanish and how it can enhance communication with Spanish-speaking patients.

In the realm of healthcare, expressing necessity and making recommendations are daily occurrences. The subjunctive mood is particularly valuable in these scenarios. For instance, consider the phrase "*Es importante que el paciente tome su medicamento,*" which translates to "It's important that the patient takes his medication." In this context, the subjunctive mood conveys a sense of necessity. The healthcare professional is emphasizing the importance of the patient taking their prescribed medication for their well-being.

Beyond necessity, the subjunctive mood is also employed to express wishes and give advice. For instance, you might encounter the phrase "*Es mejor que descanses,*" which can be translated as "It is better if you rest." In this case, the use of the subjunctive mood signifies that resting is advisable for the patient's benefit. It offers a gentle and caring way to make recommendations, acknowledging that the patient has agency in the decision.

Understanding the subtleties of the subjunctive mood in Spanish can significantly enhance communication with Spanish-speaking patients, especially in situations where advice, recommendations, or possible treatment outcomes need to be conveyed. When healthcare professionals can navigate the subjunctive mood effectively, they not only communicate medical information accurately but also demonstrate a level of linguistic proficiency that fosters trust and rapport with their patients.

So, let's start by analyzing the conjugation of the verb "*ser*" (to be) in the present subjunctive for the grammatical personals that we learned back in Chapter 1:

Pronoun	Conjugation (ser)
Yo	*sea*
Tú	*seas*
Él/Ella/Usted	*sea*
Nosotros	*seamos*
Vosotros	*seáis*
Ellos/Ellas/Ustedes	*sean*

Examples:

- *Es fundamental que el médico sea comprensivo y respetuoso al tratar a los pacientes de diferentes culturas.*

324 | SOL MANCILLA

- (It is essential that the doctor be understanding and respectful when treating patients from different cultures.)
- *Recomiendo que ustedes **sean** conscientes de las creencias culturales de sus pacientes para brindarles una atención más sensible.*
- (I recommend that you all be aware of your patient's cultural beliefs to provide more sensitive care.)
- *Es importante que los profesionales de la salud **seamos** capaces de comunicarnos efectivamente en español médico para garantizar un cuidado de calidad.*
- (It is important that healthcare professionals be capable of communicating effectively in medical Spanish to ensure quality care.)

Here's a chart with the conjugations of the verb "***estar***" (to be) in the past, present, and future simple subjunctive tenses:

Subject pronoun	Past simple subjunctive	Present simple subjunctive	Future simple subjunctive
Yo	*estuviera*	*esté*	*estuviere*
Tú	*estuvieras*	*estés*	*estuvieres*
Él/Ella/Usted	*estuviera*	*esté*	*estuviere*
Nosotros(as)	*estuviéramos*	*estemos*	*estuviéremos*
Vosotros(as)	*estuvierais*	*estéis*	*estuviereis*
Ellos/Ellas/Ustedes	*estuvieran*	*estén*	*estuvieren*

Examples:

- *Quería que él* **estuviera** *en la reunión.* (I wanted him to be at the meeting.) -Past simple subjunctive.
- *Es importante que tú* **estés** *tranquilo.* (It's important that you are calm.) -Present simple subjunctive.
- *Si no vienen, llamaré a un familiar para que* **estuviere** *presente.* (If they don't come, I will call a relative so that they will be present.) -Future simple subjunctive.

As we previously mentioned, the present subjunctive tense in Spanish is a valuable tool for healthcare professionals when they need to express advice and recommendations or discuss possible treatment outcomes. This tense allows for more nuanced communication, conveying necessity, doubt, or possibility. Let's explore this further with examples and charts featuring the conjugations of the verbs "*tener*" (to have) and "*necesitar*" (to need) in the present subjunctive.

The present subjunctive of "*tener*" can be used to express the necessity of something. For example:

- *Es importante que el paciente* **tenga** *una dieta equilibrada.* (It's important that the patient has a balanced diet.)
- *El médico recomienda que ustedes* **tengan** *cuidado con el sol.* (The doctor recommends that you all be careful with the sun.)

Here's the chart with the conjugations of "*tener*" in the present subjunctive:

Pronoun	Conjugation
Yo	*tenga*
Tú	*tengas*
Él/Ella/Usted	*tenga*
Nosotros(as)	*tengamos*
Vosotros(as)	*tengáis*
Ellos/Ellas/ Ustedes	*tengan*

The present subjunctive of "*necesitar*" can be used to discuss the patient's need for specific treatments or care. For example:

- *No creo que el paciente **necesite** que el médico le dé una receta.* (I don't think the patient needs the doctor to give them a prescription.)
- *Es probable que **necesitemos** hacer un examen de orina.* (We may need to do a urine test.)

Here's the chart with the conjugations of "*necesitar*" in the present subjunctive:

Pronoun	Conjugation
Yo	necesite
Tú	necesites
Él/Ella/Usted	necesite
Nosotros(as)	necesitemos
Vosotros(as)	necesitéis
Ellos/Ellas/Ustedes	necesiten

NAVIGATING COMPOUND TENSES

In Spanish, compound tenses are a crucial aspect of effective communication, especially when discussing healthcare matters. These tenses are used to indicate actions that have a specific relationship with other actions in terms of time and completion. Understanding and using compound tenses correctly can greatly enhance your ability to convey complex medical information to Spanish-speaking patients.

The **compound past perfect** tense is frequently used in healthcare conversations to describe actions that have occurred in the past and are still relevant to the present moment. It is formed by combining the auxiliary verb "*haber*" (to have) with the past participle of the main verb. Here's an example:

- "*El paciente **ha** tomado su medicamento*" (The patient **has** taken his medication).

In this sentence, "*ha tomado*" (has taken) is in the past perfect tense. It indicates that the action of taking medication happened at some point in the past, and its effects or relevance continues into the present. This tense is valuable when discussing a patient's recent medical history, ensuring that you convey the continuity of their actions or treatments.

The **compound future perfect** tense is used to express the assumption or speculation that an action will have been completed by a specific future time or event. This tense can be particularly useful when discussing treatment plans, expected outcomes, or predictions related to a patient's health. It is formed by combining the future tense of the auxiliary verb "***haber***" with the past participle of the main verb. Here's an example:

- "*El paciente **habrá** terminado su tratamiento en un mes*" (The patient **will** have finished his treatment in a month).

In this sentence, "*habrá terminado*" (will have finished) is in the future perfect tense. It suggests that, based on current information or planning, the patient's treatment is expected to be completed in the future. This can help healthcare professionals communicate effectively about long-term treatment goals and anticipated results.

Mastering compound tenses in Spanish allows healthcare professionals to convey intricate medical information with precision and clarity. For example, you can use the past perfect tense to describe a patient's detailed medical history, providing a comprehensive understanding of their prior health conditions and treatments. On the other hand, the future perfect tense enables you to discuss treatment plans and expected outcomes, giving patients a clear picture of what lies ahead in their healthcare journey.

Here's a chart that conjugates the verb "*ser*" in the past and future compound tenses in Spanish, along with sentences related to a clinical environment using each tense:

Verb "ser" (to be)	Past perfect tense	Future perfect tense
Yo	he sido	habré sido
Tú	has sido	habrás sido
Él/Ella/Usted	ha sido	habrá sido
Nosotros(as)	hemos sido	habremos sido
Vosotros(as)	habéis sido	habréis sido
Ellos/Ellas/Ustedes	han sido	habrán sido

Examples:

- *En el pasado, el paciente **ha** sido muy activo antes de su lesión.* (In the past, the patient has been very active before his injury). -Compound past perfect
- *Hasta el momento, el diagnóstico **ha** sido ambiguo, pero seguiremos investigando.* (So far, the diagnosis has been ambiguous, but we will continue investigating). - Compound past perfect

- *Para la próxima cita, el paciente **habrá** sido sometido a una serie de pruebas adicionales.* (By the next appointment, the patient will have undergone a series of additional tests). - Compound future perfect

Let's see other verbs conjugated in the **compound past perfect** tense:

Pronouns	Verb "tomar" (to take)	Verb "descansar" (to rest)	Verb "recuperar" (to recover)
Yo	he tomado	he descansado	he recuperado
Tú	has tomado	has descansado	has recuperado
Él/Ella/Usted	ha tomado	ha descansado	ha recuperado
Nosotros(as)	hemos tomado	hemos descansado	hemos recuperado
Vosotros(as)	habéis tomado	habéis descansado	habéis recuperado
Ellos/Ellas/Ustedes	han tomado	han descansado	han recuperado

Examples:

- Yo **he** *tomado* la temperatura del paciente cada dos horas. (I have taken the patient's temperature every two hours).
- El médico pregunta si el paciente **ha** *descansado* al menos ocho horas antes de la cirugía. (The doctor asks if the patient has rested at least eight hours before surgery).
- Después de la operación, el paciente **ha** *recuperado* la conciencia gradualmente. (After the surgery, the patient has gradually regained consciousness).

It can be challenging to differentiate between a compound tense and another. Here's a chart with the pronouns and the conjugation for the past and future compound tenses for the verb "*necesitar*" (to need) so you can better notice the difference. Don't forget to check the use examples below:

Pronouns	Past perfect (I had needed)	Future perfect (I will have needed)
Yo	he necesitado	habré necesitado
Tú	has necesitado	habrás necesitado
Él/Ella/Usted	ha necesitado	habrá necesitado
Nosotros(as)	hemos necesitado	habremos necesitado
Vosotros(as)	habéis necesitado	habréis necesitado
Ellos/Ellas/Ustedes	han necesitado	habrán necesitado

Examples:

- *Antes de la cirugía, el paciente* **ha** *necesitado tomar medicamentos para reducir el dolor.* (Before the surgery, the patient had needed to take medication to reduce the pain). -Compound past perfect
- *Durante su recuperación, el paciente* **ha** *necesitado atención médica constante.* (During their recovery, the patient had needed constant medical care). -Compound past perfect
- *Después de la cirugía, el paciente* **habrá** *necesitado tiempo para descansar y recuperarse por completo.* (After the surgery, the patient will have needed time to rest and fully recover). -Compound future perfect

DECODING IDIOMATIC EXPRESSIONS

Idiomatic expressions, known as *"expresiones idiomáticas"* in Spanish, are phrases that carry a figurative meaning that is often different from their literal translation. They are a distinctive feature of the Spanish language and are used extensively in everyday conversations. Understanding these expressions is crucial for effective communication, especially in a healthcare setting.

Being aware of these expressions is essential for healthcare professionals when interacting with Spanish-speaking patients. These expressions often carry nuanced meanings that can significantly affect the context of a conversation. Here's how understanding idiomatic expressions can enhance patient communication:

- Misinterpreting idiomatic expressions can lead to misunderstandings in healthcare discussions. For example, if a patient says, *"Me duele el brazo, pero no es la gran cosa"* (My arm hurts, but it's not the big thing), they might downplay their symptoms.
- Familiarity with idiomatic expressions can foster a stronger rapport with Spanish-speaking patients. When healthcare professionals acknowledge and use these expressions appropriately, it conveys a level of cultural competence and empathy. Patients may feel more comfortable and understood when their healthcare provider recognizes and responds to their use of idiomatic language.

Here are some of the most common idiomatic expressions in Spanish, along with their meanings:

- "*Estar en las nubes*:" To be daydreaming or not paying attention, often used when someone is mentally distracted.
- "*Más sano que una pera*:" To be in very good health, indicating robust well-being.
- "*Echar agua al mar*:" To do something pointless or futile, similar to "casting pearls before swine."
- "*Costar un ojo de la cara*:" To cost an arm and a leg, indicating something is very expensive.
- "*Estar en las últimas*:" To be on one's last legs, typically referring to someone who is very ill or exhausted.
- "*Meter la pata*:" To put one's foot in one's mouth or make a big mistake.
- "*Dar en el clavo*:" To hit the nail on the head, meaning to be exactly right about something.
- "*Ser pan comido*:" To be a piece of cake, indicating that something is very easy.
- "*Tener mala leche*:" To be in a bad mood or have a bad attitude.
- "*Estar en el séptimo cielo*:" To be in seventh heaven, signifying extreme happiness or bliss.
- "*Buscarle la quinta pata al gato*:" To look for trouble where there isn't any, similar to "making a mountain out of a molehill."

ADVANCED MEDICAL TERMINOLOGIES

In this section, we will explore a wide range of complex medical terms in Spanish. You'll encounter specific illnesses and conditions, as well as advanced medical procedures and treatments. These terms are essential for healthcare professionals who want to provide precise and accurate information to Spanish-speaking patients. Understanding these advanced medical terminologies will enable you to navigate intricate medical discussions and offer comprehensive care.

Here is a chart with common diseases and chronic conditions encountered in healthcare settings, along with their translations and pronunciation in Spanish:

English term	Spanish translation	Pronunciation
Anemia	*Anemia*	ah-neh-mee-ah
Asthma Attack	*Ataque de asma*	ah-tah-keh deh ahs-mah
Celiac Disease	*Enfermedad celíaca*	ehn-fehr-meh-dahd seh-lee-ah-kah
Chronic Obstructive Pulmonary Disease (COPD)	*Enfermedad Pulmonar Obstructiva Crónica (EPOC)*	ehn-fer-meh-dahd pool-moh-nahr ohbs-troock-tee-vah kroh-nee-kah
Glaucoma	*Glaucoma*	glaw-koh-mah
Hepatitis	*Hepatitis*	eh-pah-tee-tees
High Cholesterol	*Colesterol alto*	koh-leh-ste-rol al-toh
Hemorrhoids	*Hemorroides*	eh-moh-roy-dehs
Hypoglycemia	*Hipoglucemia*	ee-poh-gloo-seh-mee-ah
Hypothyroidism	*Hipotiroidismo*	ee-poh-tee-roh-ee-dees-moh
Kidney Stones	*Cálculos renales*	kahl-koo-lohs reh-nah-lehs
Lupus	*Lupus*	loo-poos
Multiple Sclerosis	*Esclerosis Múltiple*	ehs-kleh-roh-sees mool-tee-pleh
Osteoarthritis	*Osteoartritis*	ohs-teh-oh-ar-tree-teess
Osteosarcoma	*Osteosarcoma*	ohs-teh-oh-sar-koh-mah
Parkinson's Disease	*Enfermedad de Parkinson*	ehn-fehr-meh-dahd deh pahr-keen-sohn
Psoriasis	*Psoriasis*	soh-ree-ah-sis
Rheumatoid Arthritis	*Artritis reumatoide*	ahr-tree-teess reh-oo-mah-tow-ee-deh
Tuberculosis	*Tuberculosis*	too-ber-koo-loh-sis
Varicose Veins	*Venas varicosas*	veh-nahs vah-ree-koh-sahs

Next, here is the chart with the medical equipment terms:

English term	Spanish translation	Pronunciation
Ambulance	Ambulancia	ahm-boo-lahn-syah
Bedpan	Orinal	oh-ree-nahl
Blood Bag	Bolsa de sangre	bohl-sah deh sahn-greh
Blood Pressure Monitor	Monitor de presión arterial	moh-nee-tor deh preh-see-on ahr-teh-ryahl
Crutches	Muletas	moo-leh-tahs
Defibrillator	Desfibrilador	des-fee-bree-lah-dohr
EKG Machine	Máquina de electrocardiograma	mah-kee-nah deh eh-lehk-troh-kar-dee-oh-grah-mah
Electrocardiogram (ECG) Machine	Máquina de electrocardiograma (ECG)	mah-kee-nah deh eh-lehk-troh-kar-dee-oh-grah-mah
Electroencephalogram (EEG) Machine	Máquina de electroencefalograma (EEG)	mah-kee-nah deh eh-lehk-troh-en-sef-ah-loh-grah-mah
Echocardiogram (Echo) Machine	Máquina de ecocardiograma (Echo)	mah-kee-nah deh eh-koh-kar-dee-oh-grah-mah
Glucometer	Glucómetro	gloo-koh-meh-tro
IV (Intravenous) Drip	Goteo intravenoso	goh-teh-oh een-trah-veh-noh-soh
IV Catheter	Catéter intravenoso	kah-teh-tehr een-trah-veh-noh-soh
IV Pole	Soporte para suero	soh-por-teh pah-rah sweh-roh
MRI Machine	Máquina de resonancia magnética	mah-kee-nah deh reh-soh-nahn-see-ah mahg-neh-tee-kah
Nebulizer	Nebulizador	neh-boo-lee-sah-dor
Ophthalmoscope	Oftalmoscopio	ohf-tahl-moh-sko-pee-oh
Otoscope	Otoscopio	oh-toh-sko-pee-oh
Pulse Oximeter	Oxímetro de pulso	ok-see-meh-tro deh pool-soh
Scales	Báscula	bahs-koo-lah
Scalpel	Bisturí	bee-stoo-ree

Sphygmomanometer	Esfigmomanómetro	es-feeg-moh-mah-noh-meh-tro
Stethoscope	Estetoscopio	ehs-teh-tohs-koh-pee-oh
Suction Machine	Máquina de succión	mah-kee-nah deh sook-see-ohn
Surgical Gloves	Guantes quirúrgicos	gwahn-tehs kee-roor-hee-kohs
Thermometer	Termómetro	ter-moh-meh-tro
Tourniquet	Torniquete	tohr-nee-ket-eh
Ultrasound Machine	Máquina de ultrasonido	mah-kee-nah deh ool-trah-soh-nee-doh
Ventilator	Ventilador	ven-tee-lah-dor
Wheelchair	Silla de ruedas	see-yah deh roo-eh-dahs
X-ray Machine	Máquina de rayos X	mah-kee-nah deh rah-yos eh-kees

These terms are now sorted alphabetically to facilitate easy reference for healthcare professionals working with Spanish-speaking patients.

Examples:

- El paciente fue diagnosticado con diabetes, por lo que necesita llevar un **glucómetro** *para controlar su nivel de azúcar en la sangre.* (The patient was diagnosed with diabetes, so he needs to carry a glucometer to monitor his blood sugar level.)
- *La paciente sufrió una lesión grave y se realizó una* **resonancia magnética** *para evaluar el alcance de los daños en su columna vertebral.* (The patient suffered a serious injury, and an MRI was performed to assess the extent of damage to her spine.)
- *Después de la cirugía, se le colocó un* **catéter intravenoso** *para administrar los medicamentos de manera continua.* (After

surgery, an IV catheter was placed to administer medications continuously.)

- *El paciente experimenta una* **hipertensión** *persistente que requiere medicación para controlar su presión arterial alta.* (The patient experiences persistent hypertension that requires medication to control his high blood pressure.)

- *La* **radiografía** *mostró una fractura en el húmero, lo que explicaría el dolor intenso en el brazo.* (The X-ray revealed a fracture in the humerus, which would explain the intense pain in the arm.)

- *La* **cirugía laparoscópica** *se realizó con éxito para extirpar el* **apéndice inflamado** *y aliviar los síntomas del paciente.* (The laparoscopic surgery was performed successfully to remove the inflamed appendix and relieve the patient's symptoms.)

EXERCISES AND PRACTICE

A. Use the present perfect subjunctive of the verb "*ver*" (to see) to fill in the blanks:

1. *El médico insiste en que el paciente no* _____*(ver) más sangrado.*
2. (The doctor insists that the patient doesn't see any more bleeding.)
3. *Espero que tú* _____*(ver) mejoras en tu salud pronto.*
4. (I hope that you see improvements in your health soon.)

Answers:

1. *vea*
2. *veas*

B. Complete the sentences using the present perfect subjunctive of "*entender*" (to understand):

1. *Es fundamental que los profesionales de la salud* _____*(entender) las necesidades de los pacientes.*
2. (It is essential that healthcare professionals understand the patients' needs.)
3. *Dudo que el padre* _____*(entender) la gravedad de la situación.*
4. (I doubt that the father understands the seriousness of the situation.)

Answers:

1. *entiendan*
2. *entienda*

C. Consider the conjugation of the verb "*haber*" (to have) in the present perfect subjunctive and complete the sentences below:

Pronoun	Conjugation (present subjunctive)
Yo	haya
Tú	hayas
Él/Ella	haya
Nosotros/Nosotras	hayamos
Vosotros/Vosotras	hayáis
Ellos/Ellas	hayan

1. *Quiero que tú* _____ (1) *entendido las instrucciones.* (I want you to have understood the instructions.)
2. *Es necesario que él* _____ (2) *completado el tratamiento.* (It is necessary for him to have completed the treatment.)
3. *Espero que ustedes* _____ (3) *tomado la medicina a tiempo.* (I hope that you all have taken the medicine on time.)

Answers:

1. *hayas*
2. *haya*
3. *hayan*

D. Consider the conjugation of the verb "*saber*" (to know) in the past, present, and future simple subjunctive tenses and complete the sentences below:

1. *Es importante que tú* _____ *la respuesta correcta* (present subjunctive of "*saber*").
2. *Quería que él* _____ *la verdad* (past subjunctive of "*saber*").
3. *Es crucial que ellos* _____ *qué hacer en caso de emergencia* (present subjunctive of "*saber*").

Answers:

1. *Sepas*
2. *Supiera/supiese*
3. *Sepan*

E. Read the following dialogue and identify the compound tenses of the bold verbs:

*Doctor (D): Buenos días, señor García. Veo que **ha** tenido (1) algunos síntomas preocupantes recientemente.* _____

*Paciente (P): Sí, doctor. **He** sentido (2) fatiga y dolores en el pecho.*

_____

*D: Comprendo su preocupación. Primero, **ha** tenido (3) problemas cardíacos en el pasado, ¿verdad?* _____

P: Sí, tuve un infarto hace algunos años.

*D: Entiendo. Hemos realizado algunos estudios y **ha** salido (4) un poco de irregularidad en su ritmo cardíaco. Esto podría estar relacionado con su historial médico.* _____

P: ¿Qué debo hacer al respecto, doctor?

*D: Para su diagnóstico, **hemos** decidido hacer (5) un electrocardiograma adicional y le recomendamos realizarlo lo antes posible. Esto nos permitirá entender mejor su situación.* _____

P: Está bien, doctor. ¿Y cuál es el tratamiento?

*D: Una vez tengamos los resultados, **habremos** determinado (6) la mejor opción de tratamiento para usted. Deberá seguir una dieta y un régimen de ejercicios específicos, además de **haber** tomado (7) medicamentos para controlar su ritmo cardíaco.* _____,

_____

*P: Gracias, doctor. **Habré** seguido (8) sus instrucciones al pie de la letra.*

_____

D: Eso es muy importante, señor García. Estamos aquí para ayudarlo a mejorar su salud y calidad de vida.

Answers:

1. Past perfect
2. Past perfect
3. Past perfect
4. Past perfect
5. Past perfect
6. Future perfect
7. Future perfect

8. Future perfect

Translation:

D: Good morning, Mr. García. I see that you've *experienced* (1) some concerning symptoms recently.

P: Yes, doctor. I've *felt* (2) fatigue and chest pains.

D: I understand your concern. First, you've *had* (3) heart problems in the past, correct?

P: Yes, I had a heart attack a few years ago.

D: I understand. We've conducted some tests, and there **has** *been* (4) a bit of irregularity in your heart rhythm. This could be related to your medical history.

P: What should I do about it, doctor?

D: For your diagnosis, we've *decided* to perform (5) an additional electrocardiogram, and we recommend that you have it done as soon as possible. This will allow us to better understand your situation.

P: Alright, doctor. And what is the treatment?

D: Once we have the results, we **will have** *determined* (6) the best treatment option for you. You'll need to follow a specific diet and exercise regimen, in addition to **having** *taken* (7) medications to control your heart rhythm.

P: Thank you, doctor. I **will have** *followed* (8) your instructions to the letter.

D: That's very important, Mr. García. We're here to help you improve your health and quality of life.

7

CONVERSING SPANISH: A CAREER CATALYST

In the final chapter of our journey through the world of medical Spanish, we delve into a realm beyond the clinical setting. While the previous chapters equipped you with the linguistic skills and cultural insights necessary for providing exceptional patient care, this chapter unveils a new dimension: how mastering Spanish can elevate your healthcare career.

We explore how your proficiency in Spanish can be a career catalyst, opening doors to new opportunities and enhancing your professional profile. In a world that increasingly values cultural diversity and effective communication, your ability to converse in Spanish can be a valuable asset.

LANGUAGE SKILLS AS A CAREER BOOSTER

Being bilingual is an incredible asset in today's interconnected world, and when it comes to the healthcare industry, this proficiency becomes even more valuable. In this chapter, we explore the myriad opportunities that mastering Spanish can unlock in the healthcare sector. From improved earning potential to enhanced patient-provider relationships, your ability to converse in Spanish can truly be a career catalyst.

One of the most compelling reasons to embrace bilingualism, especially in a language as widely spoken as Spanish, is the economic advantage it brings. According to a study, bilingual workers tend to earn between 5% to 20% more per hour than their monolingual counterparts (Shin & Alba, 2009). This wage premium is a testament to the high demand for bilingual professionals across various industries, including healthcare.

In the realm of healthcare, where effective communication is paramount, bilingual healthcare professionals are sought after. Hospitals, clinics, and medical practices often prioritize candidates who can bridge language gaps and connect with diverse patient populations. This not only opens doors to higher-paying positions but also contributes to greater job satisfaction.

The ability to communicate with a larger patient population broadens your career horizons in healthcare. In an increasingly diverse society, healthcare providers must cater to patients from various cultural and linguistic backgrounds. Your proficiency in Spanish allows you to serve as a crucial link between healthcare services and Spanish-speaking patients.

Beyond the clinical setting, your language skills can be a valuable asset in administrative roles, healthcare management, or public health initiatives that target Spanish-speaking communities.

Effective communication is at the heart of quality healthcare, and being bilingual can significantly enhance the patient-provider relationship. When patients can communicate directly with their healthcare providers in their preferred language, it fosters trust and rapport.

Moreover, bilingual healthcare professionals can offer a more personalized and efficient healthcare experience. Eliminating the need for interpreters streamlines the communication process, reducing the risk of miscommunication and ensuring that crucial medical information is accurately conveyed.

Your Spanish language skills are a valuable asset that should be prominently featured on your resume. When applying for healthcare positions, whether as a nurse, physician, pharmacist, or any other role, consider including your language proficiency in the "skills" section of your CV.

For instance, you might write, "proficient in medical Spanish, with experience providing healthcare to Spanish-speaking patients." This concise statement immediately communicates your ability to interact with a diverse patient population and can capture the attention of potential employers.

During job interviews, take the opportunity to showcase how your Spanish skills have positively impacted your work. Share specific examples of how effective communication in Spanish has led to improved patient care, better outcomes, or enhanced collaboration with colleagues.

If you've undergone formal training or hold certifications in Spanish language proficiency, such as those from the American

Council on the Teaching of Foreign Languages (ACTFL), be sure to include them on your resume. Certifications provide tangible evidence of your language proficiency and can set you apart from other candidates.

Additionally, certifications from reputable organizations like ACTFL are widely recognized and respected in the industry. They demonstrate your commitment to maintaining high language standards and can be a powerful endorsement of your language skills.

Building strong relationships with colleagues and patients is crucial in healthcare. Embracing Spanish in your professional interactions can be a meaningful way to connect with Spanish-speaking colleagues and foster a more inclusive workplace environment.

Simple gestures like greeting your Spanish-speaking colleagues in their native language can go a long way in building camaraderie and showing respect for their culture. Engaging in casual conversations or using Spanish during team meetings can help strengthen bonds and create a more cohesive healthcare team.

Furthermore, attending networking events or professional conferences specifically designed for Spanish-speaking healthcare professionals can be a game-changer for your career. These events provide a unique platform to practice your Spanish language skills, exchange insights with peers, and expand your professional network.

As you progress in your career, it's essential to continue expanding your medical vocabulary in Spanish. In previous chapters, we've explored the fundamentals of medical Spanish, from basic conversational phrases to specialized terminology. Now, let's dive deeper into the expansive world of Spanish medical terminology, where precision in communication is paramount.

Healthcare is a field rich in specialized terminology. Whether you work in primary care, surgery, pediatrics, or any other specialty, you'll encounter a myriad of medical terms specific to your area of expertise. These terms often require an in-depth understanding, not only of their meanings but also of their correct pronunciation and usage.

For example, consider the difference between "*osteoporosis*" and "*osteomalacia*." While both terms involve bone health, they represent distinct conditions with unique characteristics and treatment approaches. Mastery of such nuances is essential for accurate diagnosis and treatment.

CONTINUOUS LEARNING AND IMPROVEMENT

As a healthcare professional, the journey of mastering Spanish is a lifelong commitment. In this final section, we will explore strategies for continuous learning and improvement in Spanish, as well as turning challenges into opportunities for growth.

- Language proficiency, like any skill, requires regular practice. Embracing technology can make this easier than ever. Language learning apps such as Babbel or Rosetta Stone offer specialized courses in medical Spanish. These apps provide structured lessons and interactive exercises, allowing you to practice medical terminology and conversational skills at your own pace. Consistent practice is key to retaining and enhancing your language skills.

- Staying informed about the latest developments in your field is essential for any healthcare professional. Consider reading medical journals or articles in Spanish to expand your vocabulary and stay up-to-date with medical advancements. Websites like Medscape Español offer a wealth of medical content in Spanish. Reading specialized articles can help you grasp complex medical terminology and improve your comprehension.

- Engaging in conversation is one of the most effective ways to improve your language skills. Look for Spanish language clubs or conversation groups in your local community. Opt for groups that include other healthcare professionals so that you can practice medical Spanish within a relevant context. These interactions not only enhance your language proficiency but also provide a supportive community of like-minded individuals.

- Learning medical terminology can be challenging, but it's a hurdle that can be overcome with focused practice. If you struggle with recalling specific medical terms, consider creating flashcards. Write the medical term in Spanish on one side and its English translation on the other. Regularly reviewing these flashcards can help reinforce your memory and improve your ability to recall medical vocabulary accurately.

- Understanding the cultural nuances of your Spanish-speaking patients can be a complex task. Healthcare professionals often find it challenging to navigate the cultural differences that may impact patient care. However, this challenge can be turned into an opportunity for growth. Consider taking a course in Hispanic culture or healthcare in Hispanic communities. These courses not only deepen your cultural awareness but also equip you with valuable insights into patient expectations, beliefs, and behaviors.

- Finding time for language learning can be difficult, especially for busy healthcare professionals. However, integrating Spanish into your daily routine can make it more manageable. Utilize your commute time by listening to Spanish podcasts related to healthcare or general conversation. During breaks or downtime at work, practice speaking Spanish with colleagues who are also eager to improve their language skills. These small but consistent efforts can add up to significant progress over time.

In conclusion, mastering Spanish as a healthcare professional is an ongoing journey that requires dedication and commitment. By following these strategies for continuous learning and addressing challenges as opportunities for growth, you can enhance your language skills, provide more effective patient care, and open doors to new career opportunities. Remember that language proficiency is not a destination but a continuous process of improvement, enriching both your professional and personal life.

CONCLUSION

As we reach the end of this extensive guide, it's essential to recap the key points and encourage you, the dedicated healthcare hero, to continue your Spanish learning journey.

Throughout this book, we've explored the critical role that Spanish proficiency plays in the healthcare industry. We started with the basics, laying a strong foundation by delving into Spanish grammar rules, essential vocabulary, and common medical terminologies. We then progressed to practical applications, providing you with scenarios where your newfound Spanish skills could make a significant difference in patient care.

We ventured into specialized vocabulary tailored to different healthcare fields, ensuring that you're well-equipped to communicate effectively in your specific area of expertise. We also delved into the cultural nuances of Spanish-speaking patients, emphasizing the importance of sensitivity and patient-centered care.

For those seeking to take their Spanish skills to the next level, we delved into advanced grammar rules and complex medical terminologies, preparing you for more intricate conversations and challenging scenarios.

Our journey has highlighted the benefits of learning Spanish in the healthcare industry. By mastering this language, you unlock the ability to communicate seamlessly with Spanish-speaking patients, grasp common medical terms, and apply your knowledge practically.

Remember that the ultimate purpose of this book is to empower you to break down language barriers, enhance your communication skills, and provide the best possible care to your patients. You have embarked on a path that not only enriches your professional life but also impacts the lives of those you serve.

As we conclude, I encourage you to continue honing your Spanish skills. Consider delving further into your language journey by exploring my previous book, *Learn Spanish for Adult Beginners: Speak Confidently & Impress Your Amigos. A No-Nonsense Guide to Quickly Learn Vocabulary, Common Phrases and Master Pronunciation* (Mancilla, 2023), where you can build upon your foundational knowledge and become fluent beyond the clinical setting.

Apply what you've learned in your interactions with Spanish-speaking patients. Utilize additional resources, such as language learning apps or engaging with Spanish-speaking colleagues, for continued practice and learning.

If you found this essential guide to Spanish for healthcare professionals beneficial, I would greatly appreciate your feedback. Sharing your thoughts and experiences through reviews can be a valuable way to support fellow language learners and healthcare heroes. Your review will serve as an inspiration and encouragement for others embarking on their journey to speak Spanish confidently.

Please scan the QR code below to leave your review.

Your commitment to learning Spanish is a testament to your dedication to patient care and professional growth. Embrace this journey as an enriching experience that will positively impact your career and the lives of those you serve.

Thank you for joining me on this adventure of language and healthcare. I wish you continued success, fulfillment, and satisfaction in your healthcare profession.

Gracias por tu compromiso y empatía con las personas hispanoh-ablantes.

¡Adelante y éxito en su viaje de aprendizaje del español!

APPENDIX

In this section, you will find exercises, dialogues, more vocabulary, and grammar reinforcements to continue practicing your Spanish and take it to the next level. Take your time doing the exercises and try not to consult the answers unless necessary or to double-check.

Have fun learning this wonderful language!

A. Complete the following sentences with the appropriate definite article (el, la, los, or las) in Spanish:

1. _____ *obstetra examina a la paciente.* (masculine)
2. _____ *bebés nacieron sanos.* (masculine)
3. _____ *parto fue complicado pero exitoso.*
4. _____ *enfermeros están cuidando a las pacientes.*
5. _____ *ginecólogo brinda atención especializada.*
6. _____ *mujeres embarazadas necesitan controles regulares.*

7. _____ *cirujano realizó una cesárea.*
8. _____ *pacientes están en la sala de espera.*
   (femenine)
9. _____ *recién nacido está en perfecto estado.*
10. _____ *parteras ayudaron en el parto en casa.*
11. _____ *ecografía reveló el género del bebé.*
12. _____ *pacientes deben seguir las indicaciones*
    médicas.
13. _____ *anestesista administró la epidural.*
    (masculine)
14. _____ *madres primerizas a veces tienen ansiedad.*
15. _____ *médico realiza exámenes de rutina.*

Translation:

1. The obstetrician examines the patient.
2. The babies were born healthy.
3. The childbirth was challenging but successful.
4. The nurses are taking care of the patients.
5. The gynecologist provides specialized care.
6. Pregnant women need regular check-ups.
7. The surgeon performed a cesarean section.
8. The patients are in the waiting room.
9. The newborn is in perfect condition.
10. The midwives assisted with the home birth.
11. The ultrasound revealed the baby's gender.
12. Patients must follow medical instructions.
13. The anesthesiologist administered the epidural.
14. First-time mothers sometimes experience anxiety.
15. The doctor conducts routine exams.

Answers:

1. *El*
2. *Los*
3. *El*
4. *Los*
5. *El*
6. *Las*
7. *El*
8. *Las*
9. *El*
10. *Las*
11. *La*
12. *Los*
13. *El*
14. *Las*
15. *El*

B. Fill in the blanks with the appropriate personal pronouns (yo, tú, él, ella, nosotros, vosotros, ellos, ellas) in Spanish:

1. _____ *soy el anestesiólogo encargado de la cirugía.*
2. _____ *debes administrar la anestesia de manera precisa.*
3. _____ *tiene experiencia en anestesiología pediátrica.*
4. _____ *estudia las reacciones a los anestésicos.*
5. _____ *trabajamos en equipo en el quirófano.*
6. _____ *debéis estar preparados para emergencias.*
7. _____ *investigan nuevas técnicas anestésicas.*
8. _____ *cuidan a los pacientes antes de la cirugía.*

9. _____ *explicaré el procedimiento a la paciente.*

10. _____ *monitorizas constantemente la presión arterial.*

11. _____ *debe calcular la dosis adecuada del anestésico.*

12. _____ *prefiere la anestesia regional.*

13. _____ *nos preocupamos por el bienestar del paciente.*

14. _____ *tenéis experiencia en anestesia obstétrica.*

15. _____ *acompañan al paciente a la sala de recuperación.*

Answers:

1. *Yo*
2. *Tú*
3. *Él/Ella*
4. *Él/Ella*
5. *Nosotros/as*
6. *Vosotros/as*
7. *Ellos/Ellas*
8. *Ellos/Ellas*
9. *Yo*
10. *Tú*
11. *Él/Ella*
12. *Él/Ella*
13. *Nosotros/as*
14. *Vosotros/as*
15. *Ellos/Ellas*

Translation:

1. I am the anesthesiologist in charge of the surgery.
2. You must administer anesthesia accurately.
3. He/She has experience in pediatric anesthesiology.
4. He/She studies reactions to anesthetics.
5. We work as a team in the operating room.
6. You all must be prepared for emergencies.
7. They research new anesthesia techniques.
8. They take care of patients before surgery.
9. I will explain the procedure to the patient.
10. You continuously monitor blood pressure.
11. He/She must calculate the appropriate dose of the anesthetic.
12. He/She prefers regional anesthesia.
13. We care about the patient's well-being.
14. You all have experience in obstetric anesthesia.
15. They accompany the patient to the recovery room.

C. Complete the following sentences by conjugating the given verbs in the specified tense (present simple, past perfect simple, or future simple) in Spanish:

1. (*Hablar*; Presente Simple) *El paciente* _____ *con el terapeuta sobre sus preocupaciones.*
2. (*Comprender*; Pasado Perfecto Simple) *El psicólogo* _____ *las razones detrás de su ansiedad.*
3. (*Resolver*; Futuro Simple) *El tratamiento* _____ *los problemas emocionales del paciente.*

4. (*Analizar*; Presente Simple) *Los expertos* _____ *los síntomas del trastorno.*

5. (*Superar*; Pasado Perfecto Simple) *El paciente* _____ *sus traumas pasados.*

6. (*Evaluar*; Futuro Simple) *El psiquiatra* _____ *el progreso del tratamiento.*

7. (*Observar*; Presente Simple) *Los investigadores* _____ *el comportamiento del grupo de control.*

8. (*Diagnosticar*; Pasado Perfecto Simple) *El médico* _____ *el trastorno en una etapa temprana.*

9. (*Mejorar*; Futuro Simple) *La terapia* _____ *la calidad de vida del paciente.*

10. (*Tratar*; Presente Simple) *Los profesionales* _____ *a personas con trastornos mentales.*

11. (*Entender*; Pasado Perfecto Simple) *Ella* _____ *la causa de su depresión.*

12. (*Prevenir*; Futuro Simple) *La medida* _____ *futuros episodios de ansiedad.*

13. (*Diagnosticar*; Presente Simple) *Los especialistas* _____ *trastornos neuropsiquiátricos.*

14. (*Controlar*; Pasado Perfecto Simple) *El paciente* _____ *sus impulsos agresivos.*

15. (*Guiar*; Futuro Simple) *El terapeuta* _____ *al paciente hacia la recuperación.*

Answers:

1. *Habla*
2. *Comprendió*
3. *Resolverá*

4. *Analizan*

5. *Superó*

6. *Evaluará*

7. *Observan*

8. *Diagnosticó*

9. *Mejorará*

10. *Tratan*

11. *Entendió*

12. *Prevenirá*

13. *Diagnostican*

14. *Controló*

15. *Guiará*

Translation:

1. The patient speaks with the therapist about their concerns.
2. The psychologist understood the reasons behind their anxiety.
3. The treatment will resolve the patient's emotional issues.
4. The experts analyze the symptoms of the disorder.
5. The patient overcame his/her past trauma.
6. The psychiatrist will evaluate the progress of the treatment.
7. The researchers observe the behavior of the control group.
8. The doctor diagnosed the disorder at an early stage.
9. The therapy will improve the patient's quality of life.
10. Professionals treat people with mental disorders.
11. She understood the cause of her depression.

12. The measure will prevent future episodes of anxiety.

13. Specialists diagnose neuropsychiatric disorders.

14. The patient controlled his aggressive impulses.

15. The therapist will guide the patient toward recovery.

D. Look at the bold verbs and identify in which tense and for which grammatical person they are conjugated:

Cirujano (C): Buenos días, doctor. Tenemos a la paciente García en la sala de operaciones. **Prepararon***(1) todo el equipo necesario para la cirugía de reconstrucción de la fractura de fémur.*

Anestesiólogo (A): Buenos días, doctor. Me **alegra***(2) escuchar eso. Antes de proceder, ¿***ha revisado***(3) la historia clínica de la paciente?*

C: Sí, la **revisé***(4). La paciente* **sufrió***(5) un accidente en moto hace tres días y* **presentó***(6) múltiples fracturas. Su estado general* **ha sido***(7) estable hasta el momento, pero* **necesitamos***(8) realizar esta cirugía para evitar complicaciones a largo plazo.*

A: Entiendo. ¿La paciente **ha recibido***(9) algún tipo de medicación preoperatoria?*

C: No, aún no. **Hablé***(10) con ella antes de la cirugía para asegurarme de que no* **comió***(11) alimentos ni tomó líquidos en las últimas ocho horas, como se recomienda.*

A: Perfecto. **Voy***(12) a administrar la anestesia general. Una vez que la paciente esté dormida, ¿cuánto tiempo* **durará***(13) la cirugía?*

C: Estimamos que la cirugía **llevará***(14) aproximadamente tres horas. Durante ese tiempo,* **debemos***(15) realizar la reducción de la fractura y fijar la placa y los tornillos para asegurar la estabilidad del hueso.*

A: Entendido, doctor. Me **aseguraré**(16) *de mantener a la paciente bajo anestesia de manera segura durante todo el procedimiento.*

C: Excelente. Una vez que **haya finalizado**(17) *la cirugía,* **necesitaremos**(18) *su colaboración para despertar a la paciente y monitorizar su recuperación en la sala de recuperación postoperatoria.*

A: Por supuesto, **estaré**(19) *allí para supervisar la transición de la paciente del estado de sedación al de conciencia. Después* **continuaremos**(20) *evaluando su estado y administrando el manejo del dolor según sea necesario.*

Translation:

Surgeon (S): Good morning, doctor. We have patient García in the operating room. They prepared all the necessary equipment for the femur fracture reconstruction surgery.

Anesthesiologist (A): Good morning, doctor. I'm glad to hear that. Before proceeding, have you reviewed(3) the patient's medical history?

S: Yes, I reviewed it. The patient suffered a motorcycle accident three days ago and she presented multiple fractures. Her general condition has been stable, but we need to perform this surgery to avoid long-term complications.

A: I understand. Has the patient received any preoperative medication?

S: No, not yet. I spoke with her before surgery to make sure she did not eat or drink in the last eight hours, as recommended.

A: Oh, perfect. I am going to administer general anesthesia. Once the patient is asleep, how long will the surgery last?

S: We estimate that the surgery will take approximately three hours. During that time, we must perform fracture reduction and fix the plate and screws to ensure the stability of the bone.

A: Understood, doctor. I will make sure to keep the patient safely under anesthesia throughout the procedure.

S: Excellent. Once the surgery has been completed, we will need your collaboration to wake up the patient and monitor her recovery in the post-operative recovery room.

A: Of course, I will be there to supervise the patient's transition from anesthesia to consciousness. Afterward, we will continue to assess her condition and administer pain management as necessary.

Answers:

[*Infinitive verb*]: [*tense*]; [*Personal pronoun*]

1. **Preparar**: *Pasado perfecto simple; Ellos/as*
2. **Alegrar**: *Presente; Yo*
3. **Revisar**: *Pasado perfecto compuesto; Usted*
4. **Revisar**: *Pasado perfecto simple; Yo*
5. **Sufrir**: *Pasado perfecto simple; Ella*
6. **Presentar**: *Pasado perfecto simple; Ella*
7. **Ser**: *Pasado perfecto compuesto; Ella*
8. **Necesitar**: *Presente; Nosotros/as*
9. **Recibir**: *Pasado perfecto compuesto; Ella*
10. **Hablar**: *Pasado perfecto simple; Yo*

11. **Comer:** *Pasado perfecto simple; Ella*
12. **Ir:** *Presente; Yo*
13. **Durar:** *Futuro Simple; Ella (la cirugía)*
14. **Llevar:** *Futuro Simple; Ella (la cirugía)*
15. **Deber:** *Presente; Nosotros/as*
16. **Asegurar:** *Futuro Simple; Yo*
17. **Finalizar:** *Pasado perfecto compuesto; Ella (la cirugía)*
18. **Necesitar:** *Futuro Simple; Nosotros/as*
19. **Estar:** *Futuro Simple; Yo*
20. **Continuar:** *Futuro Simple; Nosotros/as*

E. Read the following dialogue and translate the bold words:

Niño (N): ¡Hola, doctor! **Mamá**(1) *me dijo que necesito* **anteojos**(2) *porque tengo* **miopía**(3) *y* **astigmatismo**(4)*, pero no entiendo qué significa eso. ¿Puede explicármelo?*

Oftalmólogo (O): ¡Hola! Claro que puedo explicártelo. La miopía y el astigmatismo son dos **problemas de la visión**(5)*. Comencemos por la miopía. La miopía significa que puedes ver claramente los* **objetos cercanos**(6)*, como un libro, pero tienes* **dificultades**(7) *para ver* **cosas lejanas**(8)*, como la pizarra en la escuela.*

N: Ah, entiendo. ¿Y qué es el astigmatismo?

O: Bueno, el astigmatismo es un poco diferente. En el astigmatismo, la forma de tu **ojo**(9) *no es perfectamente* **redonda**(10)*, como una pelota. En cambio, puede ser más como un balón de rugby. Esto hace que la luz que entra en tu ojo no se* **enfoque**(11) *adecuadamente en un solo punto de la* **retina**(12)*, y eso provoca* **visión borrosa**(13) *tanto de cerca como de lejos.*

N: Gracias, doctor. ¿Cómo saben que tengo estos problemas? ¿Qué hacen en la **consulta**(14)?

O: Para saber si tienes miopía y astigmatismo, te haremos un **examen visual completo**(15). *Usaremos una máquina llamada* **refractómetro**(16) *para medir la forma en que la luz se dobla cuando pasa por tu ojo. También puedes mirar a través de una serie de* **lentes**(17) *mientras lees* **letras**(18) *en una* **carta de Snellen**(19) *para determinar cuál te ayuda a ver más claramente.*

N: ¿Y los anteojos ayudarán a que pueda ver mejor?

O: Exacto, los anteojos corregirán estos problemas. Para la miopía, los lentes tendrán una forma específica para ayudar a que los rayos de luz se enfoquen adecuadamente en tu retina, permitiéndote ver objetos lejanos con claridad. En el caso del astigmatismo, los lentes serán especialmente diseñados para enderezar la luz y mejorar tu visión tanto de cerca como de lejos.

N: Gracias por explicármelo, doctor. ¿Cómo serán los anteojos?

O: Los anteojos serán diseñados para que se adapten a tu **prescripción**(20) *exacta. Pueden ser de diferentes estilos y colores, ¡así que podrás elegir los que más te gusten!*

Answers:

1. Mom
2. Glasses
3. Myopia
4. Astigmatism
5. Vision problems
6. Near objects

7. Difficulties
8. Distant objects
9. Eye
10. Round
11. Focus
12. Retina
13. Blurry vision
14. Consultation
15. Comprehensive visual examination
16. Refractometer
17. Lenses
18. Letters
19. Snellen chart
20. Prescription

Translation:

Child (C): Hello, doctor! Mom told me I need glasses because I have myopia and astigmatism, but I don't understand what that means. Can you explain it to me?

Ophthalmologist (O): Hello! Of course, I can explain it to you. Myopia and astigmatism are two vision problems. Let's start with myopia. Myopia means that you can see objects up close, like a book, clearly, but you have difficulties seeing distant things, like the chalkboard at school.

C: Ah, I see. And what is astigmatism?

O: Well, astigmatism is a bit different. In astigmatism, the shape of your eye is not perfectly round, like a ball. Instead, it can be more like a rugby ball. This causes the light entering your eye not to focus properly on a single point of the retina, and that causes blurry vision both up close and far away.

C: Thank you, doctor. How do they know I have these problems? What do they do during the consultation?

O: To find out if you have myopia and astigmatism, we will perform a comprehensive visual examination. We will use a machine called a refractometer to measure how light bends when it passes through your eye. You will also look through a series of lenses while reading letters on a Snellen chart to determine which one helps you see more clearly.

C: Will glasses help me see better?

O: Exactly. Glasses will correct these problems. For myopia, the lenses will have a specific shape to help the light rays focus properly on your retina, allowing you to see distant objects clearly. In the case of astigmatism, the lenses will be specially designed to straighten the light and improve your vision both up close and far away.

C: Thank you for explaining it, doctor. What will the glasses look like?

O: The glasses will be designed to fit your exact prescription. They can come in different styles and colors, so you can choose the ones you like the most!

F. Read the following scenarios and write down (in Spanish) below what you would do as a healthcare professional:

Escenario 1: Un paciente en la sala de emergencias presenta síntomas de un infarto de miocardio, como dolor en el pecho intenso y opresión.

_____

_____

Escenario 2: Una mujer embarazada llega al hospital con contracciones regulares y fuertes.

_____

_____

Escenario 3: En la unidad de cuidados intensivos, un paciente está experimentando una crisis epiléptica.

_____

_____

Escenario 4: Un niño es traído a la sala de urgencias con una fiebre alta y dificultad para respirar.

_____

_____

Escenario 5: Un paciente mayor es admitido en el hospital con síntomas de un posible derrame cerebral.

_____

_____

Translation:

Scenario 1: A patient in the emergency room presents with symptoms of a heart attack, such as severe chest pain and tightness.

Scenario 2: A pregnant woman arrives at the hospital with regular, strong contractions.

Scenario 3: In the intensive care unit, a patient is experiencing a seizure.

Scenario 4: A child is brought to the emergency room with a high fever and difficulty breathing.

Scenario 5: An elderly patient is admitted to the hospital with symptoms of a possible stroke.

Potential Answers:

1. *Debes tomar medidas rápidas para estabilizar al paciente, administrar aspirina y preparar para una posible angioplastia.* (You must take quick measures to stabilize the patient, administer aspirin, and prepare for possible angioplasty.)
2. *Como profesional de la salud, debes evaluar su estado y ayudar en el proceso de parto, brindando apoyo y monitorizando al bebé y a la madre.* (As a health professional, you must evaluate her condition and help in the birth process, providing support and monitoring the baby and the mother.)
3. *Tu tarea es administrar medicamentos antiepilépticos y tomar medidas para evitar lesiones durante la convulsión.* (Your task is to administer antiepileptic medications and take steps to prevent injury during the seizure.)
4. *Como profesional de la salud, debes realizar una evaluación completa, tomar muestras para pruebas y administrar tratamiento para la enfermedad respiratoria.* (As a healthcare professional, you must perform a complete evaluation, collect samples for testing, and administer treatment for the respiratory illness.)

5. *Tu responsabilidad es realizar una evaluación neurológica rápida, tomar una tomografía computarizada cerebral y administrar tratamiento para minimizar el daño cerebral.* (Your responsibility is to perform a quick neurological evaluation, take a brain CT scan, and administer treatment to minimize brain damage.)

G. Observe the following diagram and match the diagnosis with the appropriate treatment:

Diagnósticos:

1. *El paciente presenta síntomas de fiebre alta, dolor de garganta y fatiga. Tras un examen físico y análisis de sangre, se confirma que padece una infección viral aguda. No se observan signos de infección bacteriana.*
2. *Este paciente tiene antecedentes de alergias estacionales y presenta síntomas de congestión nasal, picazón en los ojos y estornudos frecuentes. Después de una evaluación clínica, se confirma una reacción alérgica.*
3. *El paciente ha experimentado dolor abdominal, diarrea y fiebre durante varios días. Después de exámenes de laboratorio y una revisión completa de la historia médica, se establece el diagnóstico de gastroenteritis bacteriana.*

Tratamientos:

A.

- *Reposo en cama para permitir que el cuerpo se recupere.*
- *Hidratación constante con agua, caldos claros y bebidas electrolíticas.*
- *Antibióticos recetados específicos para tratar la infección bacteriana.*
- *Evitar alimentos grasos, picantes y lácteos hasta que los síntomas mejoren.*

B.

- *Descanso absoluto en casa.*
- *Hidratación adecuada con agua y bebidas isotónicas.*
- *Analgésicos de venta libre para reducir la fiebre y aliviar el dolor de garganta.*
- *Evitar el contacto cercano con otras personas para prevenir la propagación de la infección.*

C.

- *Antihistamínicos de venta libre para aliviar la congestión nasal y la picazón en los ojos.*
- *Uso de un humidificador en el dormitorio para mantener la humedad adecuada.*
- *Evitar la exposición a alérgenos conocidos, como el polen.*
- *Consulta de seguimiento si los síntomas persisten o empeoran.*

Answers:

1-B

2-C

3-A

Translations:

Diagnosis:

1. The patient presents symptoms of high fever, sore throat, and fatigue. After a physical examination and blood tests, it is confirmed that he suffers from an acute viral infection. No signs of bacterial infection are observed.
2. This patient has a history of seasonal allergies and presents with symptoms of nasal congestion, itchy eyes, and frequent sneezing. After clinical evaluation, an allergic reaction is confirmed.
3. The patient has experienced abdominal pain, diarrhea, and fever for several days. After laboratory tests and a complete review of the medical history, the diagnosis of bacterial gastroenteritis is established.

Treatments:

A.

- Bed rest to allow the body to recover.
- Constant hydration with water, clear broths, and electrolyte drinks.

- Specifically prescribed antibiotics to treat the bacterial infection.
- Avoid fatty, spicy, and dairy foods until symptoms improve.

B.

- Absolute rest at home.
- Adequate hydration with water and isotonic drinks.
- Over-the-counter pain relievers to reduce fever and relieve sore throat.
- Avoid close contact with other people to prevent the spread of infection.

C.

- Over-the-counter antihistamines to relieve nasal congestion and itchy eyes.
- Using a humidifier in the bedroom to maintain proper humidity.
- Avoid exposure to known allergens, such as pollen.
- Follow-up visit if symptoms persist or worsen.

H. Read the following text where a healthcare professional communicates her diagnosis to an oncological patient compassionately and efficiently, and answer (in Spanish) the questions below:

Juana, antes que nada, quiero que sepas que estamos aquí para apoyarte en cada paso de este camino. Comprendemos que este es un momento difícil para ti y estamos comprometidos a brindarte la mejor atención posible. Quiero comenzar explicándote tu diagnóstico y el plan de tratamiento que hemos diseñado para ti.

Después de realizar una serie de pruebas y análisis médicos, hemos confirmado que tienes un Linfoma no Hodgkin en estadio III. Este es un tipo de cáncer que afecta el sistema linfático, que es parte fundamental de tu sistema inmunológico. La buena noticia es que hemos identificado esto a tiempo, y con el tratamiento adecuado, tenemos la esperanza de controlar y tratar tu enfermedad de manera efectiva.

El plan de tratamiento que hemos propuesto para ti es una combinación de quimioterapia e inmunoterapia, seguida de radioterapia. La quimioterapia se utiliza para eliminar las células cancerosas en tu cuerpo y reducir el tamaño del tumor. La inmunoterapia, por otro lado, es una terapia más específica que estimula tu sistema inmunológico para que pueda reconocer y atacar las células cancerosas de manera más efectiva. La radioterapia se utilizará después de la quimioterapia e inmunoterapia para tratar áreas específicas donde el cáncer pueda persistir.

Sabemos que esta información puede ser abrumadora, pero estamos aquí para responder a todas tus preguntas y preocupaciones. Estas a salvo con nosotros.

Questions:

1. *¿Cuál es el diagnóstico médico de Juana?* (What is Juana's medical diagnosis?)
   _____
   _____

2. *¿Cuál es el objetivo de la quimioterapia en el plan de tratamiento?* (What is the goal of chemotherapy in the treatment plan?)
   _____
   _____

3. *¿Qué función tiene la inmunoterapia en el tratamiento de Juana?* (What is the role of immunotherapy in Juana's treatment?)
   _____
   _____

4. *¿Cuándo se utilizará la radioterapia en el plan de tratamiento?* (When will radiation therapy be used in the treatment plan?)
   _____
   _____

5. *¿Qué se enfatiza en cuanto a la comunicación con Juana durante esta conversación?* (What is emphasized regarding communication with Juana during this conversation?)
   _____
   _____

Translation of the text:

Juana, first of all, I want you to know that we are here to support you every step of the way. We understand that this is a difficult time for you and we are committed to providing you with the best care possible. I want to start by explaining your diagnosis and the treatment plan we have designed for you.

After performing a series of tests and medical analyses, we have confirmed that you have stage III non-Hodgkin lymphoma. This is a type of cancer that affects the lymphatic system, which is a fundamental part of your immune system. The good news is that we have identified this early, and with the right treatment, we hope to control and treat your disease effectively.

The treatment plan we have proposed for you is a combination of chemotherapy and immunotherapy, followed by radiotherapy. Chemotherapy is used to kill cancer cells in your body and shrink the tumor. Immunotherapy, on the other hand, is a more specific therapy that stimulates your immune system so it can recognize and attack cancer cells more effectively. Radiation therapy will be used after chemotherapy and immunotherapy to treat specific areas where cancer may persist.

We know this information can be overwhelming, but we are here to answer all your questions and concerns. You are safe with us.

I. Observe and learn the following vocabulary about hours of the day and days of the week and their proper usage when prescribing medication to patients:

Horas del día **(Hours of the day)**

- 12:00 a.m. - *Medianoche*
- 1:00 a.m. - *La una de la madrugada*
- 2:00 a.m. - *Las dos de la madrugada*
- 3:00 a.m. - *Las tres de la madrugada*
- 4:00 a.m. - *Las cuatro de la madrugada*
- 5:00 a.m. - *Las cinco de la madrugada*
- 6:00 a.m. - *Las seis de la mañana*
- 7:00 a.m. - *Las siete de la mañana*
- 8:00 a.m. - *Las ocho de la mañana*
- 9:00 a.m. - *Las nueve de la mañana*
- 10:00 a.m. - *Las diez de la mañana*

- 11:00 a.m. - *Las once de la mañana*
- 12:00 p.m. - *El mediodía*
- 1:00 p.m. - *La una de la tarde*
- 2:00 p.m. - *Las dos de la tarde*
- 3:00 p.m. - *Las tres de la tarde*
- 4:00 p.m. - *Las cuatro de la tarde*
- 5:00 p.m. - *Las cinco de la tarde*
- 6:00 p.m. - *Las seis de la tarde*
- 7:00 p.m. - *Las siete de la noche*
- 8:00 p.m. - *Las ocho de la noche*
- 9:00 p.m. - *Las nueve de la noche*
- 10:00 p.m. - *Las diez de la noche*
- 11:00 p.m. - *Las once de la noche*

Now, let's include some non-o'clock times:

- 1:30 a.m. - *La una y media de la madrugada*
- 2:45 a.m. - *Las dos y cuarenta y cinco de la madrugada*
- 3:15 a.m. - *Las tres y quince de la madrugada*
- 4:20 a.m. - *Las cuatro y veinte de la madrugada*
- 5:45 a.m. - *Las cinco y cuarenta y cinco de la madrugada*
- 6:10 a.m. - *Las seis y diez de la mañana*
- 7:55 a.m. - *Las siete y cincuenta y cinco de la mañana*
- 8:45 a.m. - *Las ocho y cuarenta y cinco de la mañana*
- 9:30 a.m. - *Las nueve y treinta de la mañana*
- 10:15 a.m. - *Las diez y quince de la mañana*
- 1:45 p.m. - *La una y cuarenta y cinco de la tarde*
- 2:20 p.m. - *Las dos y veinte de la tarde*
- 3:50 p.m. - *Las tres y cincuenta de la tarde*
- 4:40 p.m. - *Las cuatro y cuarenta de la tarde*

- 5:25 p.m. - *Las cinco y veinticinco de la tarde*
- 6:05 p.m. - *Las seis y cinco de la tarde*
- 7:30 p.m. - *Las siete y treinta de la noche*
- 8:15 p.m. - *Las ocho y quince de la noche*
- 9:50 p.m. - *Las nueve y cincuenta de la noche*

Días de la semana (Days of the week)

- *Lunes*: Monday
- *Martes*: Tuesday
- *Miércoles*: Wednesday
- *Jueves*: Thursday
- *Viernes*: Friday
- *Sábado*: Saturday
- *Domingo*: Sunday

Examples of use:

- *Le recomiendo tomar este medicamento todos los días a las 8 de la mañana para controlar su presión arterial, comenzando el lunes próximo.* (I recommend taking this medication every day at 8 a.m. to control your blood pressure, starting next Monday.)
- *Los martes y jueves, a las 6 de la tarde, asegúrese de hacer ejercicio moderado durante 30 minutos para fortalecer su sistema cardiovascular.* (On Tuesdays and Thursdays at 6 p.m., be sure to do moderate exercise for 30 minutes to strengthen your cardiovascular system.)
- *A partir del miércoles, tome una pastilla antes de cada comida principal, es decir, a las 8 de la mañana, 1 de la tarde y 7 de la*

noche. (Starting Wednesday, take one pill before each main meal, that is, at 8 a.m., 1 p.m. and 7 p.m.)

- *Durante todo el fin de semana, desde el viernes hasta el domingo, recuerde descansar lo suficiente y tomar abundante líquido para ayudar en la recuperación.* (Throughout the weekend, from Friday to Sunday, remember to get plenty of rest and drink plenty of fluids to aid recovery.)

- *El próximo lunes, a las 10 de la mañana, acuda a nuestra clínica para realizar un seguimiento y ajustar su plan de tratamiento según sea necesario.* (Next Monday at 10 a.m., come to our clinic to follow up and adjust your treatment plan as needed.)

Please scan the QR code below to leave your review.

REFERENCES

Colon, I. (2019). *New research examines the economic benefits of bilingualism.* New America. http://newamerica.org/education-policy/edcentral/new-research-examines-economic-benefits-bilingualism/

Dzulkifli, M. A., & Mustafar, M. F. (2013). The influence of color on memory performance: A review. *The Malaysian Journal of Medical Sciences: MJMS, 20*(2), 3–9. https://www.ncbi.nlm.nih.gov/pmc/articles/PMC3743993/

Krist, A. H., Tong, S. T., Aycock, R. A., & Longo, D. R. (2017). Engaging patients in decision-making and behavior change to promote prevention. *Studies in Health Technology and Informatics, 240*(240), 284–302. https://www.ncbi.nlm.nih.gov/pmc/articles/PMC6996004/

Mancilla, S. (2023, July 8). *Learn Spanish for adult beginners: Speak confidently & impress your amigos. A no-nonsense guide to quickly learn vocabulary, common phrases and master pronunciation.*

Martinez, G. (2015). *Spanish in the U.S. Health Delivery System.* Instituto Cervantez | Harvard University.

McCarthy, N. (2020, December 11). *Infographic: The world's most spoken languages.* Statista Infographics. https://www.statista.com/chart/12868/the-worlds-most-spoken-languages/

Lown, B. (n.d.). *Dr. Bernard Lown.* Lown Institute. https://lowninstitute.org/about/dr-bernard-lown/

Shin, H.-J., & Alba, R. (2009). The economic value of bilingualism for Asians and Hispanics. *Sociological Forum, 24*(2), 254–275. https://www.jstor.org/stable/40210401

Thompson, S. (2021, May 27). *The U.S. has the second-largest population of spanish speakers—how to equip your brand to serve them.* Forbes. https://www.forbes.com/sites/soniathompson/2021/05/27/the-us-has-the-second-largest-population-of-spanish-speakers-how-to-equip-your-brand-to-serve-them/

www.ingramcontent.com/pod-product-compliance
Lightning Source LLC
Chambersburg PA
CBHW020431130626
46549CB00001B/77